Franc

MW01534842

# *Ketogenic*

# COOKBOOK

A STEP BY STEP BEGINNERS DIET PLAN TO RESET
YOUR METABOLISM WITH THESE EASY, HEALTHY
AND DELICIOUS LOW CARB MEALS.

## BEGINNERS GUIDE

© Copyright 2017 by Francesca Bonheur - All rights reserved.

The following eBook is reproduced below with the goal of providing information that is as accurate and as reliable as possible. Regardless, purchasing this eBook can be seen as consent to the fact that both the publisher and the author of this book are in no way experts on the topics discussed within, and that any recommendations or suggestions made herein are for entertainment purposes only. Professionals should be consulted as needed before undertaking any of the action endorsed herein.

This declaration is deemed fair and valid by both the American Bar Association and the Committee of Publishers Association and is legally binding throughout the United States.

Furthermore, the transmission, duplication or reproduction of any of the following work, including precise information, will be considered an illegal act, irrespective whether it is done electronically or in print. The legality extends to creating a secondary or tertiary copy of the work or a recorded copy and is only allowed with express written consent of the Publisher. All additional rights are reserved.

The information in the following pages is broadly considered to be a truthful and accurate account of facts, and as such any inattention, use or misuse of the information in question by the reader will render any resulting actions solely under their purview. There are no scenarios in which the publisher or the original author of this work can be in any fashion deemed liable for any hardship or damages that may befall them after undertaking information described herein.

Additionally, the information found on the following pages is intended for informational purposes only and should thus be considered, universal. As befitting its nature, the information presented is without assurance regarding its continued validity or interim quality. Trademarks that mentioned are done without written consent and can in no way be considered an endorsement from the trademark holder.

# Table of Contents

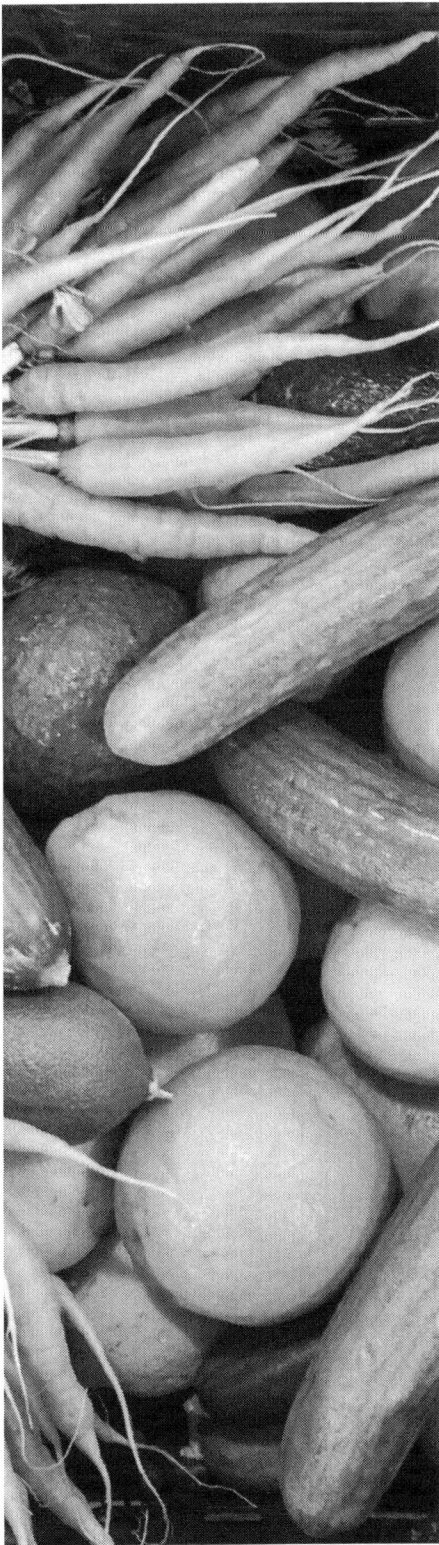

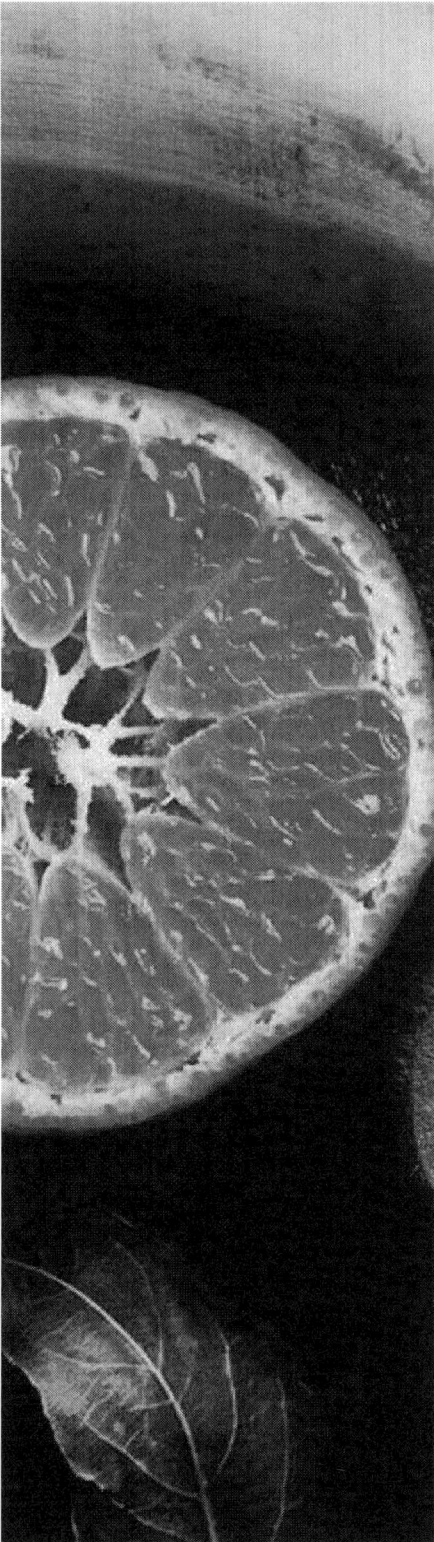

# Introduction

Congratulations on downloading your personal copy of the *Ketogenic Time to Cook Recipe Book: A step by step beginners diet plan to reset your metabolism with these easy, healthy and delicious low carb meals*. Thank you for doing so.

The following chapters will discuss some of the many delicious recipes that you can enjoy while you are doing the ketogenic diet.

You will discover how important flavors and seasonings are when you are trying to do a low-carb style of eating.

The chapters will show you the many various recipes that you can use whether it is breakfast, lunch or dinner and no matter how many people you are going to feed. The recipes are delicious.

There are plenty of books on this subject on the market, thanks again for choosing this one! Every effort was made to ensure it is full of as much useful information as possible. Please enjoy!

Congratulations on downloading your personal copy of the *Ketogenic Time to Cook Recipe Book: A step by step beginners diet plan to reset your metabolism with these easy, healthy and delicious low carb meals*. Thank you for doing so.

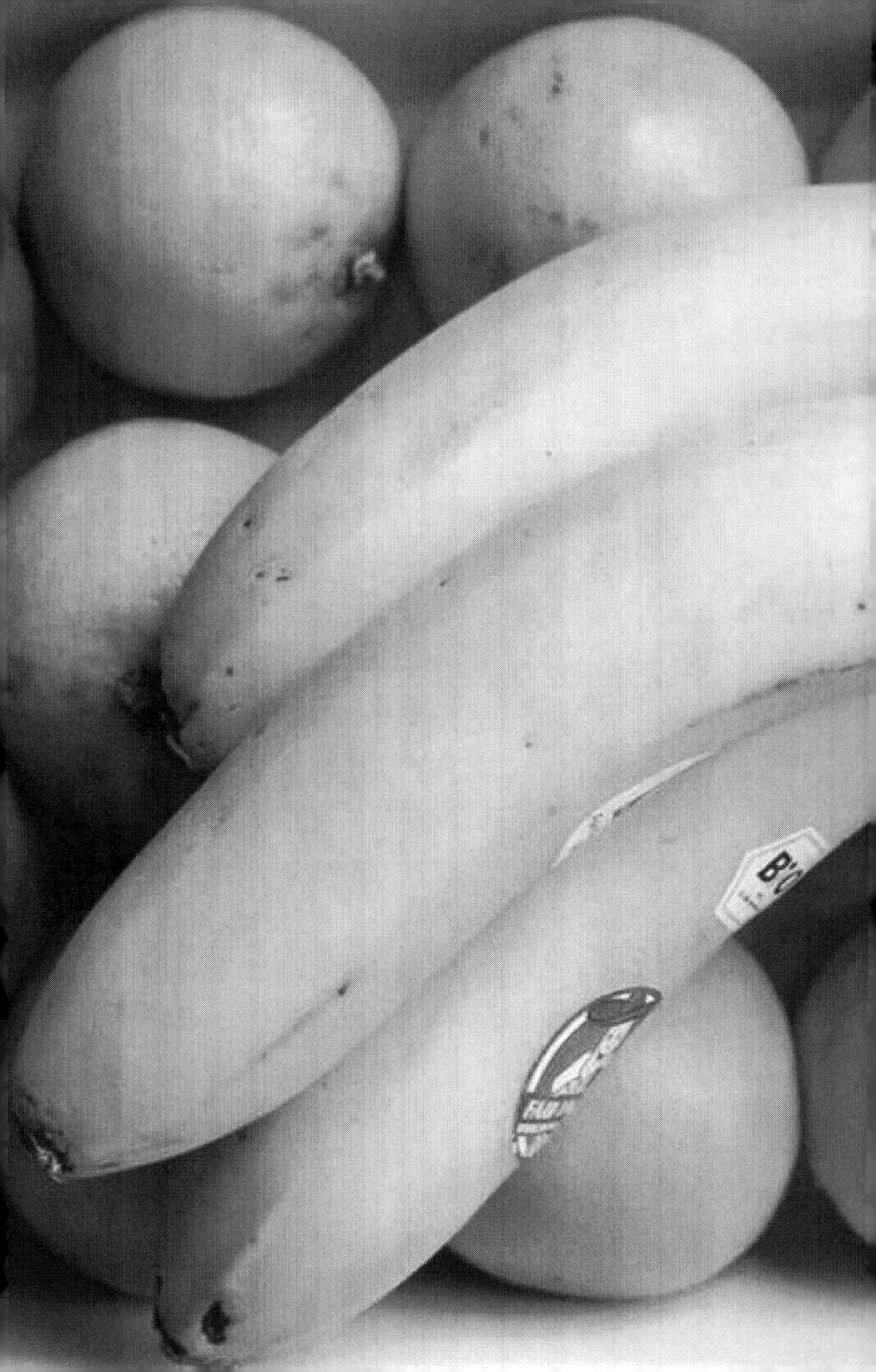

# How to Eat on the Ketogenic Diet

$\mathcal{E}$ ating according to the ketogenic diet plan is as easy as increasing the amount of fat and protein you have in your diet while also decreasing a number of carbohydrates that you consume. It is something that will enable you to lose a lot of weight and will also to help you get the most out of the different things that you are doing in your diet. When you are able to stick to the ketogenic diet plan, you will allow yourself to become as healthy as possible. Each of the recipes that are included in this book is intended to help you stick with the diet and to help you enjoy a great style of eating while simultaneously allowing you to lose weight.

## Cutting Back Won't Help

Many people have the idea that was only cutting back on the carbs that they consume will be able to help them lose the weight that they want. This false belief comes from only cutting back on the amount of the food that they eat and is not related to the carbs. To be able to actually benefit from not eating carbs, you need to be completely sure that you are not eating carbs at all. This is because you need to be able to enter into ketosis for any type of carb cutting to work truly. Without doing that, your body will not go into the fat burning mode that is required of it. You should make sure that you are not eating any carbs so that you don't have to worry about ketosis or anything that is related to ketosis. Doing each of these things is important and will allow you the chance to be completely sure that you are able to truly start losing weight.

The only way that "cutting back" will help you is if you completely cut back a number of carbs that you consume. It may benefit you to cut them slowly out but keep in mind that you will not see any weight loss in that time. The only benefit that you get from cutting back on carbs slowly is that you will not have as many carb withdrawal symptoms and they will not be as extreme as what you would have if you simply stopped eating carbs altogether. Just be sure that you are cutting back for the right reasons instead of trying to lose weight by cutting back.

## The Diet Works

What many people don't realize is that the diet works for *everyone*. Whether you have had success with low carb in the past or not, ketogenic will work for you. That is because, without unnecessary carbs, your body is able to enter into the mode that it was made for. It is a diet that is focused on natural foods and making sure that everything is alright, so it will allow you the chance to bring your body back to where it needs to be. When it comes to the ketogenic diet, you will be able to do more with it than you are with other diets.

If you do find that ketogenic is not working for you, you may want to take a look at what you are eating. There can sometimes be hidden carbs in foods that you don't even know about. This is especially true of foods that are processed because tey have sugar keeping them preserved and it can contribute to the carb count. This is one of the main reasons that it is a good idea to eat as many unprocessed foods as possible when you are doing the ketogenic diet.

## Choosing Fat

The original ketogenic diet was designed to be a low-carb and high-fat diet. This means that you will cut out the carbs that you are eating and replace them with foods that are high in fat. It is important to remember when you are doing this that fat in foods is different than fat on your body – the fat that you eat does not automatically translate to having more fat on your body. The fat that you eat is generally better for you than carbs which can mean that you will be able to get the fuel that you need when you are doing different things with that food. Just be sure that you are eating enough fat to keep you satisfied when you are trying to do ketogenic.

If you are eating enough fat and nutrition from other sources, you should not have a problem avoiding carbs while doing the ketogenic diet. You should not have too many cravings for carbs, and you really will probably not be too hungry when you are doing the diet because of the food that you *can* eat. The diet works best with high fat.

## Choosing Protein

One thing that people noticed when they were doing ketogenic diets was that they were not making the healthiest of fat choices while doing it. They were eating trans fats and foods that were not necessarily good for them while they were doing it. For this reason, the people who do the diet sometimes choose to eat protein instead of fat. This can be anything from lean protein like chicken to fatty protein like steak and other sources. Eating a diet that is rich in protein and very low in carbs will not only to help you lose weight but will also help you to gain significant muscle mass. Lean muscles will contribute to a faster metabolism and will give you the chance to be completely sure that you are getting the best nutrition possible.

It may be easier for you when you are first getting started with your diet to start out with high fat, low carb. As you progress through your diet, it may be a good idea for you to try to eat the high protein and low carb way of dieting. You will have fewer cravings when you are eating higher fat.

## Back on Track

While it is a not a good idea to get out of the habit of eating low carb, if you do get off track, you need to be completely sure that you are back on track as soon as possible. The sooner that you are able to be completely sure that you are eating low carb again, the better things will be for you. This means that you need to be completely sure that you are eating as few carbs as possible. Always try your hardest to start eating low carb again as soon as you start to get off of the regular plan.

The biggest problem with stopping eating low carb is that you will push your body out of ketosis. While it does not necessarily take a long time for you to get back into ketosis, you need to do it so that you can continue losing weight again. The low carb diet will not work if you are not able to eat low carb. You can't be in ketosis if you are still eating carbs so get back on track as soon as you can to avoid any hiccups in your weight loss program and to be completely sure that you are eating the right way.

## Substituting for Low Carb

One of the nice things about eating the ketogenic diet is that there are so many alternatives available for the typical carb-heavy foods that you eat on a regular basis. It does not take a lot of effort to replace foods, and you can even find many low-carb high-fat options available at restaurants that you would normally go to. It does not take much to be able to eat according to this plan, and you will be able to enjoy many of the same foods that you do right now – except there won't be as many carbs in the food.

While it is acceptable to eat this type of food and to try to substitute for the food, it is a good idea to eat as naturally as possible. This is one of the many benefits that come along with the ketogenic diet, and it is suggested that you do this each chance that you get. While you are working to be completely sure that you can eat low carb, you should also try to be completely sure that you are eating as naturally as possible so that you will be able to stay healthy during the diet. Low carb is a great way to eat, but low carb with natural foods is an even better way to eat.

# Breakfast Recipes

S tarting your day out with a good breakfast is one of the easiest ways that you can ensure you will not be hungry throughout the day. If you eat a breakfast that is rich in nutrients, has a high-fat content and is easy for your body to digest, you will notice that your day will be much more satisfying and you will be able to have a better day when it comes to eating. You will also notice that your time will be better overall if you Time to prep recipeare a breakfast instead of just eating an apple or something that is not filling while you are on the go.

# Raspnilla Yogurt

Serves this many: 1
Time to prep recipe: 5 minutes
Time to cook recipe: 3 minutes

## Ingredients:

- 1 domestic cup of Greek yogurt, vanilla
- 1 tsp. stevia
- ½ domestic cup of raspberries

## Directions:

1. Mix the stevia and the Greek yogurt together in a bowl. You can use a whisk to help distribute the stevia and to keep it from clumping together into large granules.

2. Put the raspberries on top of the yogurt. Add a few sprigs of mint to the top for an unexpected crisp flavor.

# Blueberry Fake Cakes

Serves this many: 2
Time to prep recipe: 5 minutes
Time to cook recipe: 10 minutes

## Ingredients:

- ½ domestic cup of almond flour
- 3 eggs
- 2 tbsp. coconut oil
- 1 tsp. stevia
- 1 tbsp. coconut oil (extra for frying)
- ¼ domestic cup of frozen blueberries

## Directions:

1. Mix your almond flour, your eggs, the coconut oil that is 2 tablespoon, and the stevia together. This works best with an electric hand mixer, but you can also do it by hand.

2. Mix the blueberries in with a spatula (fold them in).

3. Put your pan on medium heat and put your coconut oil in it (you can also use butter, but it is not as nutrient dense as the coconut oil).

4. Pour the batter into your pan just as you would usually pour pancake batter into the pan.

5. Similar to how you would do regular pancakes, wait until it starts to bubble on the top before you decide to flip the pancake.

6. Do this for each of the pancakes. It should make around 6 altogether or 3 pancakes per person.

7. You can make coconut cream or Greek yogurt to put on top of the pancakes.

# Breakfast Quiche

Serves this many: 4
Time to prep recipe: 15 minutes
Time to cook recipe: 10 minutes

## Ingredients:

- 3 eggs
- 2 pieces of bacon
- ¼ onion chopped
- 1 tbsp. coconut oil (for Time to cook recipeing)
- 1 tsp. salt
- 1 tsp. vegetable pepper
- 1 tsp. thyme

## Directions:

1.  Start out by putting your oven to 350 degrees.

2.  Fry your bacon in a pan like you would normally do. It should be crispy.

3.  Cut the bacon so that it is in small pieces.

4.  Use a whisk for the eggs.

5.  Add the onions, herbs, and spices and mix them in well. Do not use the whisk because they will clump together.

6.  Use coconut oil and rub it on the bottom and sides of a pie pan.

7.  Pour the egg mixture into the pan.

8.  You can put some shredded cheddar on top, also.

9.  Time to cook recipe for 25 – 35 minutes or until the egg is firm on the top.

# Chipotle Omelet

Serves this many: 1
Time to prep recipe: 5 minutes
Time to cook recipe: 10 minutes

## Ingredients:

- 2 eggs
- 1 slice bacon
- ¼ domestic cup of chopped green vegetable pepper
- ¼ domestic cup of chopped onion
- 1 tsp. chili
- 1 tsp. salt
- 1 tsp. vegetable pepper
- ¼ domestic cup of vegetable pepper jack cheese
- 1 tbsp. butter

## Directions:

1. Heat your pan up and Time to cook recipe your bacon.

2. Drain the bacon grease out of the pan, return to the heat.

3. Crumble your bacon so that it is in small pieces.

4. Use a whisk and beat your eggs so that the yolks are all broken up.

5. Mix the eggs and the rest of the Ingredients for Recipe together.

6. Place your butter in the pan and allow it to heat up.

7. Put the eggs with the rest of the Ingredients for Recipe in them into your frying pan that was already heated up with the bacon.

8. Allow it to Time to cook recipe for a few minutes.

9. Fold and Time to cook recipe the omelet.

# Rich and Fluffy Pancakes

Serves this many: 1
Time to prep recipe: 5 minutes
Time to cook recipe: 10 minutes

## Ingredients:

➡ ½ domestic cup of cream cheese
➡ 2 eggs
➡ 2 tsp. stevia
➡ 1 tbsp. coconut oil

## Directions:

1. Set the cream cheese out before you begin to Time to cook recipe the pancakes so that it is soft and easier for you to try to work with.

2. Mix the cream cheese, eggs and stevia together using an electric mixer.

3. Make sure that it is well combined and there are no clumps of cream cheese in it.

4. Put the coconut oil in your frying pan.

5. Heat it up over medium heat.

6. Make small medallions with the batter and pour them into the pan that you just Time to prep recipeared.

7. Wait until the pancakes begin to bubble on the top.

8. Flip them all.

9. Allow them to Time to cook recipe for only a few minutes after you have flipped them so that they don't get burnt.

10. You can serve them with butter, coconut cream or even Greek yogurt for a twist. You can also top with a few fresh berries for a pop of color and flavor that will round out your breakfast meal.

# Greek Yogurt with Coconut

Serves this many: 1
Time to prep recipe: 5 minutes
Time to cook recipe: 2 minutes

## Ingredients:

- 1 domestic cup of plain Greek yogurt
- 1 tsp. stevia
- 1 tsp. coconut extract
- 1 tsp. shredded coconut
- 2 raspberries

## Directions:

1. Mix your coconut flavoring, half of your coconut flakes, your stevia and your Greek yogurt together in a small dish. Make sure that it is well combined so that the coconut flavor will not be overpowering in the dish. This will allow you to have a better dish that you can enjoy without the extract taking over the dish.

2. Top with the rest of the shredded coconut on the top of it.

3. Put the few raspberries on top.

    *Be sure that you get the unsweetened coconut flakes.

4. Do not add more than that much coconut and raspberries. They are both on the borderline of the ketogenic diet and eating too many of either of them can kick your body out of ketosis and make losing weight much harder for you. Be sure that you are able to top them with these Ingredients for Recipe so that you can have a better type of yogurt. The burst of flavor is perfect for in the morning, and it is easy for you to eat while you are on the go.

# No Guilt Cereal

Serves this many: 1
Time to prep recipe: 5 minutes
Time to cook recipe: 1 minutes

## Ingredients:

- ½ domestic cup of coconut flakes, unsweetened, Time to cook recipeed and all natural (organic preferred)
- ¾ domestic cup of coconut milk that is unsweetened (can also substitute dairy milk)
- 1 tsp. stevia

## Directions:

1. Combine all of the Ingredients for Recipe together. Make sure that the coconut flakes are coated in the stevia to help sweeten them.

2. Mix the Ingredients for Recipe up to make a cereal-like treat.

3. Top with cinnamon or even blueberries to make the treat packed with more flavor but be sure not to include too many berries because that can push you out of ketosis.

# Fall Yogurt

Serves this many: 1
Time to prep recipe: 5 minutes
Time to cook recipe: 2 minutes

## Ingredients:

- 1 domestic cup of Greek yogurt, plain
- 1 tsp. stevia
- 1 tsp. maple extract
- 1 tbsp. walnuts

## Directions:

1. Get the walnuts ready for the recipe by chopping them either by hand or with a food processor before you start to Time to cook recipe.

2. Combine the yogurt, the stevia, and the extract and mix together so that it is all well blended together.

3. Put your chopped walnuts on top.

4. If you want to soften the walnuts slightly, put them on top the night before or even mix them with the yogurt and leave in the fridge for up to one week.

5. Makes a great breakfast for on the go.

# Flaxcakes

Serves this many: 1
Time to prep recipe: 5 minutes
Time to cook recipe: 10 minutes

## Ingredients:

- ½ domestic cup of cream cheese
- 2 eggs
- 2 tbsp. crushed flaxseed
- 2 tsp. stevia
- 1 tbsp. coconut oil

## Directions:

1. Soften the cream cheese so that it will be easier for you to work with when you are making the pancakes.

2. Mix together the cream cheese, the eggs, the flaxseed and the stevia with your hand mixer so that you will be able to be completely sure that they are combined together enough.

3. Heat up your coconut oil in a pan that is on medium heat. Do not allow it to get too hot.

4. Put the batter into the frying pan so that you can Time to cook recipe it enough.

5. When you see bubbles on the top of the pancakes, flip them over.

6. Top with any of your favorite ketogenic toppings.

7. Raspberries and whipped topping make a great, decadent treat you can enjoy in the morning for your breakfast and tastes like it might be bad for you ... but really isn't.

# Lunch Recipes

The most common time for dieters to slip up is during their lunch break. It doesn't matter if you normally eat lunch at home or at work, you should have some type of lunch Time to prep recipeared, or at least planned if you want to be able to continue to be successful with your diet. Make sure that you try each of these recipes so that you can get a new lease on lunch. The majority of the lunch recipes that are included in this book can be made ahead of time and taken to work with you so that you can make lunch hour easier on your waistline.

# Bacon Wrap

Serves this many: 2
Time to prep recipe: 5 minutes
Time to cook recipe: 5 minutes

## Ingredients:

⟹ 4 leaves romaine lettuce (large enough to wrap food up in)
⟹ 4 pieces of bacon
⟹ 1 domestic cup of spinach
⟹ 1 avocado

## Directions:

1. You should heat your skillet so that it is over the medium heat.

2. Put your bacon into the skillet and Time to cook recipe until it is crispy. It doesn't need to be over Time to cook recipeed, but crispy bacon will give you the crunch that you need to actually awaken your taste buds during the day.

3. Lay out your 4 pieces of lettuce on a clean cutting board or a countertop.

4. Cut your avocado into 2 pieces and pit it.

5. Divide it into 4 parts.

6. Slather the avocado on each of the pieces of lettuce.

7. Put the spinach down next.

8. Add the bacon last.

9. You can also put some crumbles of feta cheese on top of the bacon to add another layer of flavors to the wraps.

10. Roll the lettuce up like you would a burrito.

11. You may need to use a toothpick to keep them in place.

12. Refrigerate until you are ready to eat it to help keep the avocado from browning.

# Lunch Burger

Serves this many: 1

Time to prep recipe: 6 minutes

Time to cook recipe: 10 minutes

## Ingredients:

- 1 patty beef (you don't need to use lean but grass-fed is the best kind for you to use)
- 1 tsp. coconut oil
- 1 domestic cup of greens
- ½ avocado
- 1 tbsp. olive oil
- 1 tsp. salt
- 1 tsp. vegetable pepper

## Directions:

1. Turn your stove on so that it is heating up to the medium or the high temperature on it.

2. Put the coconut oil in the pan and allow it time to be able to melt.

3. Place your beef patty in with the coconut oil

4. Fry around 10 minutes for a medium well burger – add or subtract time depending on the doneness that you like your burgers.

5. Rinse the greens well and use a spinner to dry them.

6. Chop them up into bite sized pieces.

7. Cut your avocado until it is around the same size.

8. Mix the olive oil with the salt and the vegetable pepper.

9. Put all of the Ingredients for Recipe together except for the burger.

10. Chop up the burger into the same bite-sized pieces.

11. Toss together.

12. You can put some red onion slices on top.

13. If you would like to use a different dressing, eliminate the olive oil and only add a dressing that has no carbs or sugar.

# Dilly Egg Salad

Serves this many: 1
Time to prep recipe: 10 minutes
Time to cook recipe: 8 minutes

## Ingredients:

- 2 eggs
- 1 tbsp. mayonnaise
- 1 tsp. salt
- 1 tsp. vegetable pepper
- ½ tsp. dried dill
- 1 celery stalk
- 1 domestic cup of spinach

## Directions:

1. Get a small sauce pan and boil water in it.

2. Add your eggs and allow them to boil in the pan for around 10-12 minutes.

3. As they are boiling, wash your spinach and pat it dry or use a salad spinner to get all of the moisture out of it and keep it crunchy for as long as possible.

4. Once the eggs are done boiling, put them in an ice bath (cold water with ice in it)

5. Allow them to sit for about 5 minutes.

6. Peel them.

7. Cut them into diced chunks.

8. Add the mayonnaise, salt, vegetable pepper and dill in with the eggs.

9. Cut your celery into even smaller pieces and then add to the egg mixture.

10. Make sure that everything is mixed up well.

11. Put the egg salad on the spinach.

12. If you aren't eating within a few hours, keep the spinach and the egg salad separate.

# Cobb Salad – Keto Style

Serves this many: 1
Time to prep recipe: 10 minutes
Time to cook recipe: 10 minutes

## Ingredients:

- 1 chicken breast that has been Time to cook recipeed
- 1 piece of Time to cook recipeed bacon
- 2 domestic cup of green lettuce
- ½ avocado
- 3 cherry tomatoes
- ¼ English cucumber that is sliced
- 1 tbsp. olive oil
- 1 boiled egg diced

## Directions:

1. Wash all of your vegetables.

2. Put the lettuce into a salad spinner, dry it.

3. Cut the bacon, the chicken breast, and the lettuce into small pieces.

4. Make sure that the avocado is cut up and diced.

5. Cut the cherry tomatoes in half.

6. Peel the cucumber and dice it also. If you do not use an English cucumber, take the seeds out of it.

7. Mix all of the Ingredients for Recipe together.

8. Instead of olive oil, you can use a small amount of light Italian dressing or any other type of salad dressing that does not have carbs in it. You may want to use some mayonnaise or Greek yogurt. You can also make your own dressing using any Ingredients for Recipe that you have that do not have carbs in them and are easy to Time to prep recipeare with the salad.

21

# Bacon and Cauli Soup

Serves this many: 4
Time to prep recipe: 10 minutes
Time to cook recipe: 12 minutes

## Ingredients:

- 1 domestic cup of heavy cream
- ½ lb pieces of bacon
- 3 domestic cup of chicken stock
- 2 domestic cup of cauliflower
- 1 tsp. salt
- 1 tsp. vegetable pepper
- 1 tsp. thyme

## Directions:

1. Time to cook recipe the bacon so that it is crispy.

2. Allow it to cool and crumble into small pieces.

3. Boil water and Time to cook recipe the cauliflower in it for around 3 minutes after you have cut it into small, bite-sized pieces.

4. Mix all of the Ingredients for Recipe together into a large saucepan.

5. Allow it to Time to cook recipe for around 10 minutes.

6. Once it is done the Time to cook recipeing, use an immersion blender to be completely sure that it is all mixed up.

7. Alternatively, you can add each of the Ingredients for Recipe to a slow Time to cook recipeer and Time to cook recipe it that way – just be sure to Time to cook recipe the bacon before you do this so that you will be able to have the bacon flavor in the recipe.

8. Serve it with some chopped green onions, sour cream or even a small amount of plain yogurt to add some flavor to the recipe.

9. You can also top it with more crumbled bacon.

# Curry Chicken in Salad

Serves this many: 1
Time to prep recipe: 10 minutes
Time to cook recipe: 10 minutes

## Ingredients:

- 1 chicken breast
- 1 tbsp. coconut oil
- 3 tbsp. cream cheese
- 1 tsp. chili powder
- 1 tsp. coriander
- 1 tsp. garlic powder
- 1 tsp. onion powder

## Directions:

1. Soften the cream cheese.
2. Use a hand mixer to mix the cream cheese, the herbs, and the coconut oil together (be sure that the coconut oil is in liquid form before you try to begin the recipe).
3. Once it has all been blended together, start by cutting the chicken breast into bite sized pieces.
4. If you have not already Time to cook recipeed the chicken breast, you should do that now.
5. Add the chicken breast to the cream cheese and coconut oil mixture that you have already created.
6. Stir it up so that the chicken is well combined with the cream cheese.
7. You can serve over a bed of lettuce, eat on its own or use some of the cloud bread to make a chicken salad sandwich.
8. You don't have to use the curry mixture to get the best flavor possible – play around with other herbs and spices to a flavor that is appealing to you and your own taste buds.

# Cloud Bread

Serves this many: 8
Time to prep recipe: 5 minutes
Time to cook recipe: 3 minutes

## Ingredients:

➡ 1 box (8 ounces) cream cheese
➡ 4 eggs
➡ 1 pinch salt

## Directions:

1. Lay the cream cheese out ahead of time so that you can make sure that it is soft and you don't have to worry about the way that it is going to be too hard to be able to mix in with the rest of your Ingredients for Recipe.

2. Start out by heating up your oven to 350 degrees.

3. Mix the eggs and the salt together until the eggs begin to stiffen up and they are able to be held up by the mixer.

4. Add the cream cheese to the mixture and allow it to combine together well enough that you will not have any clumps with the cream cheese.

5. Once it is all thoroughly mixed up, you can form it into around 8 even dollops. Put it on a baking sheet that has been sprayed with Time to cook recipeing spray.

6. Put it in the oven for around 3 minutes. Use your oven light and watch it carefully because it is very easy for this type of "bread" to get burnt.

7. When it is done, substitute for any kind of bread that you would normally use.

# Ketogenic Staples

These recipes are the hallmarks for making sure that you are able to be as successful as possible on the keto diet. You can use these recipes as base dishes, side dishes or anything in between. They are ketogenic takes on classic recipes that you know and love. When you make each of these recipes, you will help to reduce the number of cravings that you have for "bad" food, and you will be able to enjoy all of the things that come along with both comfort food and ketogenic food. Make sure that you try out your favorites. The first recipe, cauliflower rice is one that you will see in both keto and not keto recipes – it is a super healthy take on a classic staple that most people use in their kitchen.

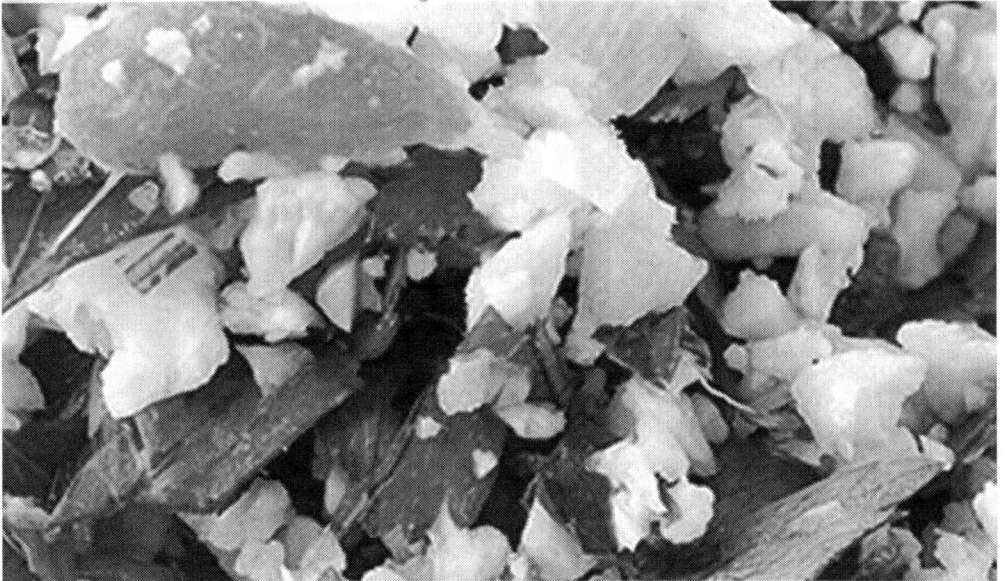

# Cauliflower Rice

Serves this many: 6
Time to prep recipe: 5 minutes
Time to cook recipe: 15 minutes

## Ingredients:

➡ 1 head cauliflower stalk discarded, cut into florets

## Directions:

1. Heat your oven and allow it to reach 425 degrees

2. Use a food processor and put the pieces of cauliflower into it.

3. Pulse for one minute or until it looks like rice. It will be in small pieces and will appear to be rice.

4. Put the cauliflower on a baking sheet and spread evenly around.

5. Bake the cauliflower for 7 ½ minutes.

6. Take the sheet out of the oven and, with an oven mitt on, spread the cauliflower around on the pan keeping it from sticking to it.

7. Put it back in the oven and Time to cook recipe for another 7 ½ minutes.

8. Store in the refrigerator for up to one week and use in any recipe that would traditionally call for you to use rice for the recipe – keto or not.

# Mashed Cauliflowers

Serves this many: 6
Time to prep recipe: 5 minutes
Time to cook recipe: 10 minutes

## Ingredients:

- 3 domestic cup of cauliflower cut into the florets
- 6 tbsp. butter
- 4 tbsp. parmesan grated
- 2 tbsp. sour cream

- 2 tbsp. cream cheese
- 2 tbsp. whipping cream
- 1 tsp. garlidomestic cup of minced
- 1 tsp. salt
- ½ tsp. vegetable pepper

## Directions:

1. Heat up a large pot that is mostly filled with water.

2. Put the cauliflower into the pot.

3. Boil it.

4. Allow it to sit in the pot while there is a rolling boil for about 5 minutes. This will help to soften the cauliflower.

5. When you put a fork into the cauliflower, and it goes in and out as easily as it would in cold butter, it is done (pro tip: this is also true for potatoes).

6. Drain the cauliflower out of the pot and put the florets into a food processor.

7. Add the rest of the Ingredients for Recipe into the food processor.

8. Pulse it for 5-second intervals.

9. Allow it to pulse for about 30 seconds.

10. All of the Ingredients for Recipe should be well combined.

11. When you are done, it should have the appearance of traditional mashed potatoes.

12. Serve with sour cream and chopped green onion.

# Cheese Pizza

Serves this many: 4
Time to prep recipe: 10 minutes
Time to cook recipe: 25 minutes

## Ingredients:

- 1 ½ domestic cup of mozzarella – shredded and divided
- ½ domestic cup of cheddar
- 1 egg
- ½ tsp. vegetable pepper
- ¼ tsp. salt
- ¼ domestic cup of sugar-free pizza sauce
- 20 slices of vegetable pepperoni

## Directions:

1. Turn your oven on and allow it to preheat until it gets to 450 degrees.
2. Mix your mozzarella with your cheddar. Add the egg and the seasonings to it and stir it very well.
3. It should resemble dough by the time that you are done mixing it, and it should stick together very well.
4. Get a 16-inch diameter pizza pan.
5. Line it with parchment paper.
6. Spread the cheese on the pan and make sure that it covers the whole bottom of it. Check for any holes in the "crust."
7. Put the pan into your oven and bake for around 15 minutes.
8. The cheese should be a golden brown color but should not be burnt.
9. Take the crust out and blot the cheese because it can tend to get greasy.
10. Put the sauce on top of the pizza.
11. Add the rest of the mozzarella cheese (1/2 c) to the crust.
12. Put the vegetable pepperoni on top.
13. Bake it for another 5 minutes or until the mozzarella on top is melted but *not* crispy.
14. Cut into 4 slices.

# Almond Bread

Serves this many: 12
Time to prep recipe: 15 minutes
Time to cook recipe: 40 minutes

## Ingredients:

- ½ domestic cup of whey protein
- 1/8 tsp. salt
- 2 tsp. baking *powder*
- ½ domestic cup of almond butter
- 4 eggs
- 1 tbsp. butter

## Directions:

1. Rub your bread pan down with the butter and make sure that it is coated on all of the sides and on the bottom.

2. Put our oven on 300 degrees and allow it to heat up.

3. Mix your whey, salt and baking powder up in a bowl and use a whisk to be completely sure that there are no clumps in it.

4. Use your hand mixer to combine the almond butter with itself. It should be creamy before you put anything else in it.

5. Add on the egg. Mix it up for about 30 seconds.

6. Add each of the rest of the eggs one each time.

7. Each time that you mix it up make sure that you are beating it up so that it is as smooth as possible.

8. It should be fluffy.

9. Fold in the whey.

10. Only mix it very gently *by hand*.

11. Using a spatula, move the batter into the pan that you just greased with butter.

12. Bake it for 30 – 40 minutes.

13. When you take out the bread, the center of it should be firm, and you should not see any movement. A knife inserted into the center will come out clean when you have done it the right way.

14. Run your knife around the outside of it so that it will come out more quickly.

15. Allow it to sit and cool down for about 10 minutes.

16. Flip the pan over onto a piece of tin foil or on a cooling rack.

17. Cover with foil or plastic wrap.

# Skinny Style Lasagna

Serves this many: 9
Time to prep recipe: 20 minutes
Time to cook recipe: 60 minutes

## Ingredients:

- 2 tbsp. olive oil
- 1 domestic cup of onion chopped
- 1 tsp. garlidomestic cup of minced
- 1 lb ground beef
- 2 domestic cup o pasta sauce
- 2 tbsp. oregano
- ¼ tsp. salt
- 1 tbsp. basil
- 2 zucchini sliced thin into 24 slices lengthwise
- 1 domestic cup of ricotta cheese in half
- 2 domestic cup of mozzarella in half
- ½ domestic cup of parmesan grated
- ¼ tsp. vegetable pepper

## Directions:

1. Put your oven on 375 degrees.

2. Use a skillet and put your olive oil into it.

3. Add the onion and the garlic to it.

4. Allow it to Time to cook recipe for a few minutes just until it becomes fragrant, and the onions start to turn clear.

5. Put your ground beef in and break it up with a spoon until it is crumbly. This should only take about 5 minutes to get to that point.

6. Put your sugar-free sauce into the mixture.

7. Allow it to simmer and then reduce it to the low setting.

31

8. Add your seasonings and anything else that you want to put into the sauce to make it more flavorful.

9. Get a square baking dish and put 6 zucchini slices in it.

10. Put the meat sauce on top. Put ¼ of a cup of ricotta on top and then sprinkle mozzarella.

11. Layer it in the same way continuously until you run out of Ingredients for Recipe. Make sure that you switch the direction that the zucchini goes in each time you make a new layer.

12. Put the rest of the cheese on the top of everything.

13. Time to cook recipe it in the oven for about 60 minutes.

14. The cheese should be brown (but not burnt) and bubble.

15. Make sure that it Time to cook recipes for about 15 minutes.

# Noodles with No Carbs

Serves this many: 8
Time to prep recipe: 30 minutes
Time to cook recipe: 90 minutes

## Ingredients:

➡ 1 large squash spaghetti variety

## Directions:

1. Take a large knife or a metal skewer and poke holes all around the spaghetti squash to allow the steam that is going to come out of it a place to escape from so that the squash does not explode while it begins to heat up in the oven.

2. Place the squash on a baking pan.

3. Heat your oven up to 350 degrees.

4. Place the squash into the oven and allow it to Time to cook recipe for about 90 minutes so that it has time to get as tender as possible.

5. Pull it out of the oven and allow it to cool until it is just slightly warm on the outside.

6. The inside will still be hot so make sure that you use oven mitts or some type of apron so that you do not get burnt.

7. Cut the spaghetti squash down the top of it, lengthwise.

8. Scoop out all of the seeds from the inside.

9. Take a fork and run it along the length of the spaghetti squash.

10. This will allow it to form thin, "spaghetti" noodles.

11. Serve it with butter, lemon juice or your favorite spaghetti sauce so that you can replace all of your traditional spaghetti pasta dishes with it.

# Dinner Recipes

inner is a time for the whole family to come together but it can feel like you're dining for one when you are trying to diet. These recipes combine the best of both worlds – healthy options for those who are doing the keto diet and delicious flavors for those who aren't. The chances are, your kids won't even know they're eating diet food and you can enjoy family dinner again ... guilt free!

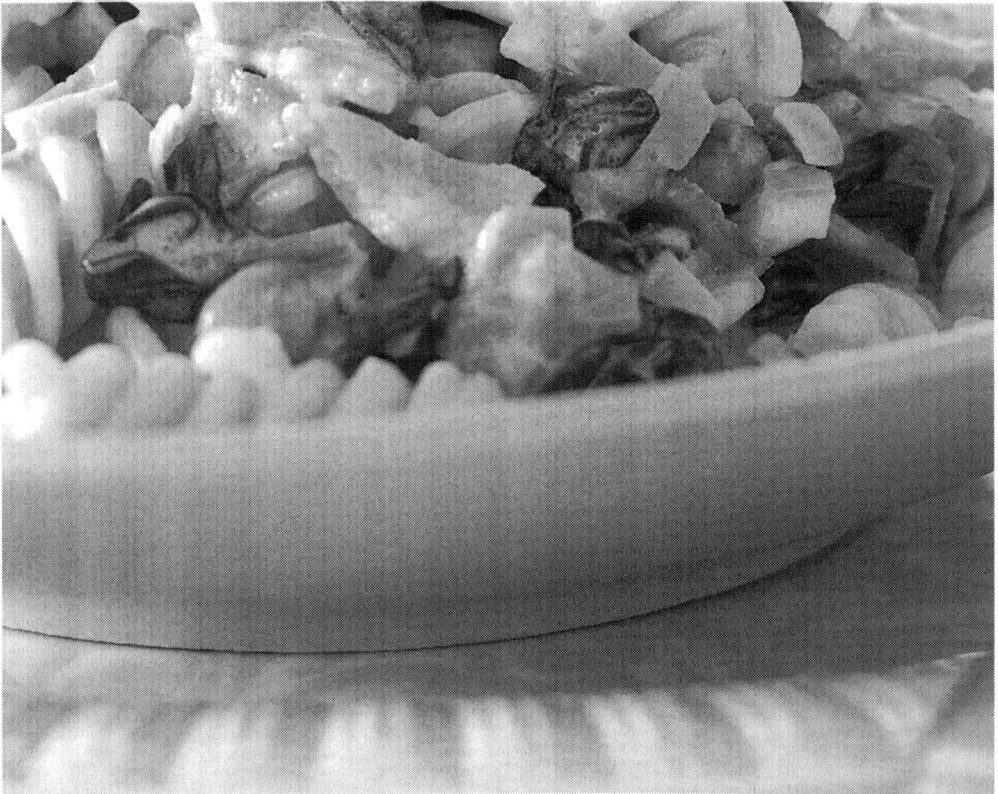

# Spinach Bacon Chicken

Serves this many: 4
Time to prep recipe: 15 minutes
Time to cook recipe: 35 minutes

## Ingredients:

- 5 slices bacon
- 2 tbsp. butter
- 1 ½ domestic cup of spinach
- 1 tsp. garlidomestic cup of minced
- ¾ domestic cup of cream cheese softened
- 1 lb chicken thighs boneless and skinless
- ¼ domestic cup of Swiss cheese shredded and divided
- ¼ tsp. salt
- ¼ tsp. vegetable pepper

## Directions:

1. Heat the oven up until it is 425 degrees.

2. Put the bacon ½ inch apart on a baking sheet.

3. Put the sheet in the oven and Time to cook recipe for 10 minutes until the bacon is crispy (you can also Time to cook recipe it in a pan on the stove).

4. Use a large skillet and make sure that the butter is melted.

5. Put the spinach and the garlic into the skillet, allow your spinach to wilt.

6. Take it out and chop the bacon into small pieces.

7. Mix these with the softened cream cheese in a large mixing bowl.

8. Lay out your chicken thighs and open them up.

9. Put the mixture into the thighs and top with a piece of Swiss cheese on each of them.

10. Close and secure them with toothpicks.

11. Rub with salt and vegetable pepper.

12. Put them in a high-walled baking dish.

13. Put the dish into the oven.

14. Time to cook recipe for around 20 minutes.

15. Always use a meat thermometer to ensure that the chicken reaches 165 degrees.

# Skinny Tenders

Serves this many: 4
Time to prep recipe: 15 minutes
Time to cook recipe: 20 minutes

## Ingredients:

- 2 eggs
- ½ domestic cup of pork rinds crushed into small pieces
- ½ domestic cup of parmesan grated
- 1 tsp. garlic powder
- 1 tsp. onion powder
- ¼ tsp. salt
- ¼ tsp. vegetable pepper
- 1 lb chicken breast boneless skinless

## Directions:

1. Start the recipe off by putting your oven at 400 degrees and allowing it to preheat.

2. Put parchment paper on your baking sheet.

3. Mix your eggs together until they are well beaten in a bowl.

4. Put the pork rinds, parmesan, and seasonings into a different bowl.

5. Put the chicken, egg bowl, pork rind bowl, and baking sheet all in a row on your counter.

6. Cut your chicken thighs so that they are only in halves.

7. Dip the chicken first in the egg and then in the pork rinds. Push it hard into the chicken so that it sticks well. Since you are working with raw chicken, you may want to consider plastic gloves (it also makes clean up easier).

8. Lay each of the pieces of chicken onto the baking sheet. If they touch, get a second baking sheet.

9. Time to cook recipe for 20 minutes.

10. Remember to always check the temperature of the chicken to ensure that it is safe for you to eat.

# Bar Chicken Wings

Serves this many: 4
Time to prep recipe: 15 minutes
Time to cook recipe: 50 minutes

## Ingredients:

- 1 tbsp. olive oil
- 1 tsp. salt
- ½ tsp. vegetable pepper
- 2 lb chicken wings
- ¼ domestic cup of hot sauce
- 1 tbsp. melted butter
- ¼ tsp. cayenne vegetable pepper
- 1 domestic cup of bleu cheese dressing (for dipping)

## Directions:

1. Heat your oven up to 400 degrees.
2. Put the olive oil, the salt, and the vegetable pepper into a big bowl.
3. Place your chicken wings in the bowl and stir them up so that they are coated in the oil.
4. Put the wings on baking sheets.
5. Put them in the oven and Time to cook recipe them until they are crispy – this should take about 50 minutes.
6. Mix the butter with the hot sauce and the cayenne together. Add a pinch of salt to this mixture.
7. When the wings are done, toss them in the sauce and allow them to sit for about 1 minute so that they are completely coated.
8. You can then divide them and serve them with the bleu cheese.
9. You can also add celery to the plate that they are on for a garnishment and to help cool down the heat that comes from the hot sauce that is in Buffalo part of the wings.

# Stuffed Chops

Serves this many: 2
Time to prep recipe: 15 minutes
Time to cook recipe: 20 minutes

## Ingredients:

- 2 tbsp. olive oil
- 1 tsp. garlidomestic cup of minced
- 3 tbsp. onion chopped fine
- 1/3 domestic cup of spinach
- 2 oz muenster cheese shredded
- 1 egg beaten
- 2 pork chops bone in
- ½ tsp. salt
- ¼ tsp. vegetable pepper

## Directions:

1. Use a large skillet that you can then put in the oven. Heat it on the medium high and put 1 teaspoon of olive oil in it. Allow it to get hot for 1 minute. Add garlic and saute it until it begins to get fragrant. Put the onion and the spinach in and lower the temperature for about three minutes.

2. Put it all in a bowl and then allow it the time to cool down.

3. Put muenster cheese and egg into it and stir so that it is all blended up and the yolk of the egg is not sticking to any one part of the mixture.

4. Heat your oven up to 375 degrees.

5. Butterfly the pork chops by cutting them through the middle. Put the spinach mixture into the pocket that you just made while you were creating the butterfly in the pork chops.

6. Don't stuff it too much because you will still need to close it up. Fold both of the sides together.

7.  Seal it with a toothpick to help keep the stuffing on the inside of it.

8.  Rub it down with the salt and the vegetable pepper.

9.  Use the same skillet and heat up another tablespoon of olive oil using the same heat. Once it is hot, lay the pork into the skillet.

10. Sear them on both sides – you should only need to do it for about 2 minutes.

11. Put the skillet into the oven.

12. Bake it for about 15 minutes.

13. Check the internal temperature for doneness – pork should always be, at least, 150 degrees. Try to stay close to that temperature because, if you go much above it, you will have pork chops that are dried out.

# Beef Brisket

Serves this many: 14

Time to prep recipe: 35 minutes

Time to cook recipe: 7 hours

## Ingredients:

- 2 tbsp. stevia
- 2 tbsp. paprika
- 1 tbsp. garlic powder
- 1 tsp. cayenne
- 1 tsp. salt
- 1 tbsp. onion powder
- 1 tbsp. vegetable pepper
- 1 tbsp. chili powder
- 8 lb beef brisket
- 2 tbsp. olive oil
- 1 ½ domestic cup of beef stock
- 1 domestic cup of onion chopped
- 1 tbsp. liquid smoke

## Directions:

*Brisket rub:*

1. Mix the stevia with your paprika, garlic powder, chili powder, cayenne vegetable pepper, salt, vegetable pepper, and onion powder. Use a small bowl to do this and make sure that they are all mixed together to be able to get all of the flavors mixed up. You can use a whisk to do this so that you will not have to worry about any of the flavors getting "stuck" together.

*Brisket:*

1. Rub down the brisket with the rub that you just made. Make sure that you take your time doing this and thoroughly coat the brisket. You should massage it to help tenderize it.

2. Heat up a large skillet with olive oil. Brown all sides of the brisket.

3. Put ½ of a cup of your beef stock into the skillet and loosen up the browned pieces of brisket.

4. Put the drippings from it into a slow Time to cook recipeer.

5. Add the rest of the stock, the onion that you chopped up and your liquid smoke. Whisk it up.

6. Put the brisket into the slow Time to cook recipeer and put some of the liquid no tops of it.

7. Time to cook recipe for 6 and a half hours on low.

# Comfort Chili

Serves this many: 12
Time to prep recipe: 30 minutes
Time to cook recipe: 2 hours

## Ingredients:

- 3 tbsp. olive oil
- 2 domestic cup of onion diced
- 3 tbsp. garlidomestic cup of minced
- 2 green vegetable peppers diced
- 2 poblanovegetable peppers diced
- 3 serrano vegetable peppers minced
- 3 jalapeno vegetable peppers diced
- 3 lb ground beef
- 1 domestic cup of tomato paste

- 2 ¼ domestic cup of crushed tomato
- 1 ½ domestic cup of diced tomatoes
- 2 domestic cup of stout beer
- 1 ½ tbsp. chili powder
- ½ tsp. paprika
- 1 tsp. salt
- 1 tsp. black vegetable pepper
- ½ tsp. cumin

## Directions:

1. Get a large stock pot and heat it up on the medium high heat setting.

2. Put your olive oil in it and then the garlic and onions. Time to cook recipe until they are tender and the onion is clear.

3. Add all of the vegetable peppers and mix for about 5 minutes until they begin to Time to cook recipe.

4. Put your ground beef in with them and make sure that you crumble it up so that it is in chunks and is broken up.

5. Once the ground beef has browned, add the tomato products and mix it up well.

6. Put the beer into the chili and allow it to come to a boil after putting the stove on high.

7. Cover it and reduce the heat. Time to cook recipe for an hour and a half.

8. Add all of the seasonings and Time to cook recipe for another 5 minutes.

9. Top with shredded cheese, sour cream or chopped green onions.

# Snack and Dessert Recipes

S nacks are a great way to keep you from getting too hungry in between meals. Eating snacks that are high in protein will allow you to be completely sure that you don't accidentally splurge on carbs. Whip up a few of these snacks ahead of time and keep them handy so that you can reach for them when you get hungry throughout the week.

The desserts that are included are great for when you just need to eat something that is sweet. They are intended to give you at treat. While you *will* probably notice that they have a "diet" taste, they can be really satisfying if you're craving carbs or sugar.

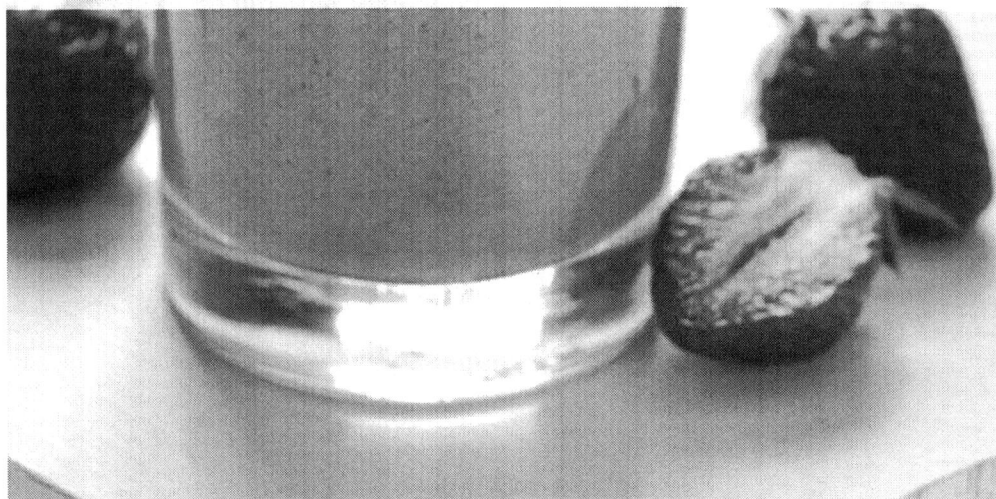

# Devil's Eggs

Serves this many: 4
Time to prep recipe: 5 minutes
Time to cook recipe: 15 minutes

## Ingredients:

- 5 eggs
- 4 slices bacon
- ½ domestic cup of mayonnaise
- 1 tbsp. mustard
- ½ tsp. paprika
- 1/8 tsp. salt
- 1/8 tsp. vegetable pepper

## Directions:

1. Fill a pot with the eggs and halfway up with water. Make sure that the eggs are covered in water and put them on the stove while bringing them to a boil over high heat.

2. Once they have started to boil, Time to cook recipe them for between 10 and 12 minutes so that they get thoroughly Time to cook recipeed through. Take the pot off and pour the eggs into an ice bath.

3. Heat up a large skillet and fry your bacon until it is crispy. Degrease the pan and allow the bacon to sit on paper towels – blot it if it is really greasy.

4. Peel the eggs and then cut them in half lengthwise.

5. Put the yolks of the eggs into a bowl and put the mayonnaise with the mustard and seasonings into the bowl. Stir it up. Cut the bacon so that it is in small pieces. Mix the bacon into the mixture also.

6. Lay the whites out in a circle and then fill the holes with the mixture. You can reserve some of the bacon and top the eggs with them and sprinkle a little more paprika on top.

7. You can also sprinkle parsley or even some small chopped green onion on the top of the eggs.

# Cheesy Chive Ham Rolls

Serves this many: 2
Time to prep recipe: 10 minutes
Time to cook recipe: 0 minutes

## Ingredients:

- 6 1/8 in thick ham slices
- 3 oz cream cheese softened
- 1 tbsp. chives chopped
- ¼ domestic cup of Monterey jack shredded
- ½ tsp. garlic powder
- ½ tsp. onion powder
- 1/8 tsp. salt
- 1/8 tsp. vegetable pepper

## Directions:

1. Put your ham rolls out on a cutting board or a plate.

2. Smear the cream cheese on the ham and make sure that each of the pieces is covered.

3. Sprinkle the chives on top of the cream cheese.

4. Add the Monterey Jack and the seasonings on top.

5. You can also just mix the seasonings with the cream cheese before you spread it on the ham if you don't want as much of a bold flavor in with the roll ups.

6. Roll each of the pieces of ham up so that they look like burritos. Secure with a toothpick if needed.

# Buffalo Dip

Serves this many: 8
Time to prep recipe: 10 minutes
Time to cook recipe: 40 minutes

## Ingredients:

- 1 stick butter
- 1 tsp. garlidomestic cup of minced
- 4 chicken thighs boneless skinless
- ¼ domestic cup of sour cream
- ¼ tsp. salt
- ¼ tsp. vegetable pepper
- ¼ tsp. cayenne
- ¼ tsp. paprika
- 1 pack cream cheese softened
- ½ domestic cup of hot sauce
- ½ domestic cup of ranch dressing
- 1 domestic cup of mozzarella shredded
- ½ domestic cup of cheddar shredded

## Directions:

1. Heat your oven up to 450 degrees.

2. Melt the butter in a large skillet and heat it on the medium high setting of your stove.

3. Add the garlic and the chicken. Time to cook recipe each of the thighs for three minutes.

4. Reduce your heat and turn it, Time to cook recipeing it for about 15 minutes. Check to be completely sure that it is at 165 degrees.

5. Move the chicken out of the pan and let it cool.

6. Shred the chicken.

7. Add sour cream with the vegetable pepper and paprika to it.

8. Put the cream cheese in a baking dish and coat the bottoms and sides of it.

9. Add the chicken to the pan.

10. Put the hot sauce and the ranch on top of the chicken. Use a spatula to get it even on the chicken.

11. Put the cheese on the top of the entire thing (you can also use bleu cheese for a different taste).

12. Time to cook recipe in the oven for about 15 minutes.

13. Allow cooling for 5 minutes.

14. Serve with celery, pork rinds or even with cloud bread.

# Dipping Kale

Serves this many: 2
Time to prep recipe: 5 minutes
Time to cook recipe: 25 minutes

## Ingredients:

- 2 domestic cup of kale – washed and trimmed
- 1 tbsp. olive oil
- ½ tsp. salt
- ½ tsp. vegetable pepper
- ½ tsp. onion powder
- ½ tsp. garlic powder

## Directions:

1. Heat your oven up to 300 degrees.

2. Put the kale and the olive oil into a large bowl (make sure that the kale is dry). Toss it in the bowl for a few minutes and make sure that all of the pieces have olive oil on them.

3. Add the seasonings to the bowl and begin to toss again. Be sure that they are all evenly coated.

4. Put parchment paper on a baking sheet.

5. Put the kale on the baking sheet.

6. Put it in the oven for 10 minutes.

7. Move the kale around the baking sheet and Time to cook recipe for another 15 minutes.

8. Give the kale a chance to cool down and get crispier before serving.

9. Goes great with any type of low or no carb dip as well as ranch dressing or even bleu cheese dressing.

# Blueberry Cheesecake Bites

Serves this many: 16 (bites)
Time to prep recipe: 60 minutes
Time to cook recipe: 0 minutes

## Ingredients:

- 4 tbsp. butter
- ½ domestic cup of cream cheese softened
- 4 tbsp. coconut oil
- 4 tbsp. whipping cream
- ¼ domestic cup of blueberries chopped
- 1 tsp. vanilla extract

## Directions:

1. Put your butter, cream cheese, and coconut oil into a bowl that is able to go into the microwave. Put it on high for 10 seconds at a time. Make sure that the coconut oil and the butter are melted.

2. When you have melted the mixture, take it out of the microwave and put the whipping cream with the blueberries into it.

3. Put everything into a food processor and pulse it for a few seconds at a time.

4. Time to prep recipeare an ice cube tray and pour the mixture into it.

5. Allow it to sit in the freezer for, at least, one hour or overnight if you have time.

# Truffles Without Guilt

Serves this many: 12
Time to prep recipe: 25 minutes
Time to cook recipe: 0 minutes

## Ingredients:

- 1 block cream cheese softened
- ½ domestic cup of stevia
- 2 tsp. coconut extract
- ½ domestic cup of shredded coconut unsweetened

## Directions:

1. Add the cream cheese and the stevia together in a mixing bowl.

2. Use a hand mixer or mix by hand to be completely sure that they are blended together well.

3. Add the coconut extract and blend well.

4. Fold in the coconut.

5. Roll spoonfuls into balls and place on a baking sheet.

6. Keep in the refrigerator.

# Personal Cake

Serves this many: 1
Time to prep recipe: 10 minutes
Time to cook recipe: 0 minutes

## Ingredients:

- 2 tbsp. cocoa powder
- 2 tbsp. stevia
- pinch salt
- 1 tbsp. whipping cream
- ½ tsp. vanilla extract
- 1 egg beaten
- ¼ tsp. baking powder

## Directions:

1. Use a large mug that you are able to put in the microwave.

2. Spray the mug with Time to cook recipeing spray.

3. In a separate bowl, mix the dry Ingredients for Recipe.

4. Add in the wet Ingredients for Recipe and stir well to combine.

5. Be sure that there are no air pockets in the mixture.

6. Put it all in the mug.

7. Heat for 1 and a half minutes on high heat.

8. Take it out and allow it to cool for about 1 minute and then eat with a spoon right out of the mug.

# Green Strawberry Smoothie

Serves this many: 2

Time to prep recipe: 10 minutes

Time to cook recipe: 0 minutes

## Ingredients:

- 1 domestic cup of ice that has already been crushed
- ½ domestic cup of almond milk
- 2 domestic cup of spinach washed and dried
- ½ domestic cup of strawberries destemmed
- 1 tbsp. coconut oil

## Directions:

1. Put half of the ice into a blender and add the rest of the Ingredients for Recipe.

2. Once it is smooth, add the rest of the ice to the mixture.

3. Be sure that it is completely smooth before you serve.

# Peanut Butter Shake

Serves this many: 2
Time to prep recipe: 10 minutes
Time to cook recipe: 0 minutes

## Ingredients:

- 1 domestic cup of ice crushed
- ¼ domestic cup of PB2 (or any other powdered peanut butter)
- ¼ domestic cup of whipping cream
- 2 tbsp. coconut oil
- 1 domestic cup of almond milk

## Directions:

1. Put half of the ice in the blender. You can do this before it is crushed and save yourself one of the steps that you would normally take.

2. Blend it up with the peanut butter powder and the cream.

3. Once it is smooth, add the oil and the milk.

4. Blend for a few more minutes.

5. When smooth, add more of the ice to it.

6. Blend for one more minute.

7. When the shake is smooth, take it out of the blender and serve it.

8. You can also add some unsweetened cocoa powder to the shake to give it a different type of flavor.

# Conclusion

Thank you for making it through to the end of the *Ketogenic Time to Cook Recipe Book: A step by step beginners diet plan to reset your metabolism with these easy, healthy and delicious low carb meals*. Let's hope it was informative and able to provide you with all of the tools you need to achieve your goals of

The next step is actually to try the recipes that are in this book – it's a very good idea to start with one of the snacks or desserts because they are *so* easy to make and can be eaten right away.

Finally, if you found this book useful in any way, a review on Amazon is always appreciated!

# Description

Dieting can be hard, but it doesn't have to. The ketogenic diet is designed to make your diet easier and to allow you the chance to have optimal health while you are shedding pounds. While the keto diet is relatively simple, it can sometimes be hard to find recipes that work with it especially when you are just getting started and don't know the right substitutions for the diet.

The Time to cook recipe book allows you the chance to be completely sure that you are getting great recipes that are low carb and high fat. They will help you to stay satisfied whether you are just starting the ketogenic diet, are in the middle of it or even if you are in the maintenance phase of it. You can benefit from each of the recipes that are included in the book. You'll be sure never to get hungry when you always have something to choose from.

All of the recipes that are included in this Time to cook recipe book are divided into convenient sections. Whether you want breakfast, lunch, dinner or just a snack, you can use the Time to cook recipe book to enjoy any of the types of meals. There are even recipes in the Time to cook recipe book that you can share with your friends who *aren't* eating a ketogenic diet. Make sure that you let them know that the recipes are great and they're healthy (even if they don't taste like it).

Read on to learn more about the ketogenic diet, how you can benefit from cutting carbs and some of the best recipes available that will help you stick to your diet. Dieters who are better Time to prep recipeared for the lifestyle they are going to enjoy will have a better chance at being able to eat that way. You can even Time to prep recipeare some of the recipes far in advance, so you just have to heat and eat.

# Francesca Bonheur

# *Ketogenic*

# COOKBOOK

RESET YOUR METABOLISM WITH THESE EASY, HEALTHY *and* DELICIOUS KETOGENIC, PALEO *and* PRESSURE COOKER...

## CHICKEN RECIPES

© Copyright 2017 Francesca Bonheur - All rights reserved.

This document is geared towards providing exact and reliable information in regards to the topic and issue covered. The publication is sold with the idea that the publisher is not required to render accounting, officially permitted, or otherwise, qualified services. If advice is necessary, legal or professional, a practiced individual in the profession should be ordered.

- From a Declaration of Principles which was accepted and approved equally by a Committee of the American Bar Association and a Committee of Publishers and Associations.

In no way is it legal to reproduce, duplicate, or transmit any part of this document in either electronic means or in printed format. Recording of this publication is strictly prohibited and any storage of this document is not allowed unless with written permission from the publisher. All rights reserved.

The information provided herein is stated to be truthful and consistent, in that any liability, in terms of inattention or otherwise, by any usage or abuse of any policies, processes, or directions contained within is the solitary and utter responsibility of the recipient reader. Under no circumstances will any legal responsibility or blame be held against the publisher for any reparation, damages, or monetary loss due to the information herein, either directly or indirectly.

Respective authors own all copyrights not held by the publisher.

The information herein is offered for informational purposes solely, and is universal as so. The presentation of the information is without contract or any type of guarantee assurance.

The trademarks that are used are without any consent, and the publication of the trademark is without permission or backing by the trademark owner. All trademarks and brands within this book are for clarifying purposes only and are the owned by the owners themselves, not affiliated with this document.

# Table of Contents

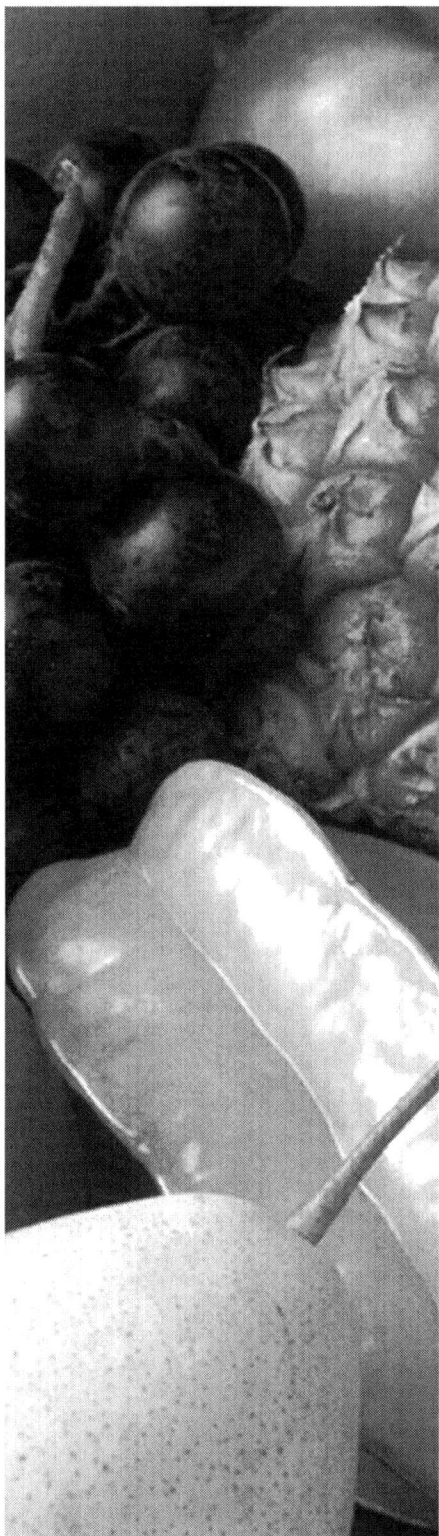

# Introduction

*I* want to thank you and congratulate you for downloading the book, "Ketogenic Cookbook: Reset Your Metabolism with these Easy, Healthy and Delicious Ketogenic, Paleo and Pressure Cooker Chicken Recipes."

Over the past few decades, new and exciting diets have popped up in the health and fitness world. Weight Watchers, the Macrobiotic Diet, Organic Food Diet, the Paleolithic Diet, and the Ketogenic diet are all examples of the countless forms and names that diets can take, but only account for a very slim percentage of all the diet choices that people have in the modern world. With so many options to choose from, and many of these options often being the new dietary trend of the week, it can be hard to determine what diet works for you personally.

This book is designed to provide you with a brief, yet comprehensive overview of two diets in particular: The Ketogenic diet and the Paleolithic diet. You may ask yourself, "why these two diets specifically? Why not some others that were mentioned in the prior list?" The answer to that is easy and comes in two major parts:

1. The Ketogenic diet and the Paleolithic diet have both been around for a long time (meaning neither is the "hot new diet" that everyone and their mothers are doing simply because it's the cool thing to do).
2. Both the Keto diet and Paleo diet have a tendency to be misunderstood by beginners looking to dip their toes. While services like Weight Watchers have large, established communities and a corporate structure, other diets (including but not limited to the Keto diet and the Paleo diet) don't have the broad, outspoken community or media presence that larger services do. It's important to know the facts before diving in, and that's just what this book will help any person do.

While this book focuses on the Keto diet and the Paleo diet specifically, it dives into even more specific territory and focuses on recipes centered on using chicken as an ingredient as well as a very special, very unique weight loss herb known as the Chrysanthemum flower that will help lose and maintain weight (as well as nearly a dozen other beneficial effects that will make weight loss and health maintenance seem like a breeze!).

Thanks again for downloading this book, I hope you enjoy it!

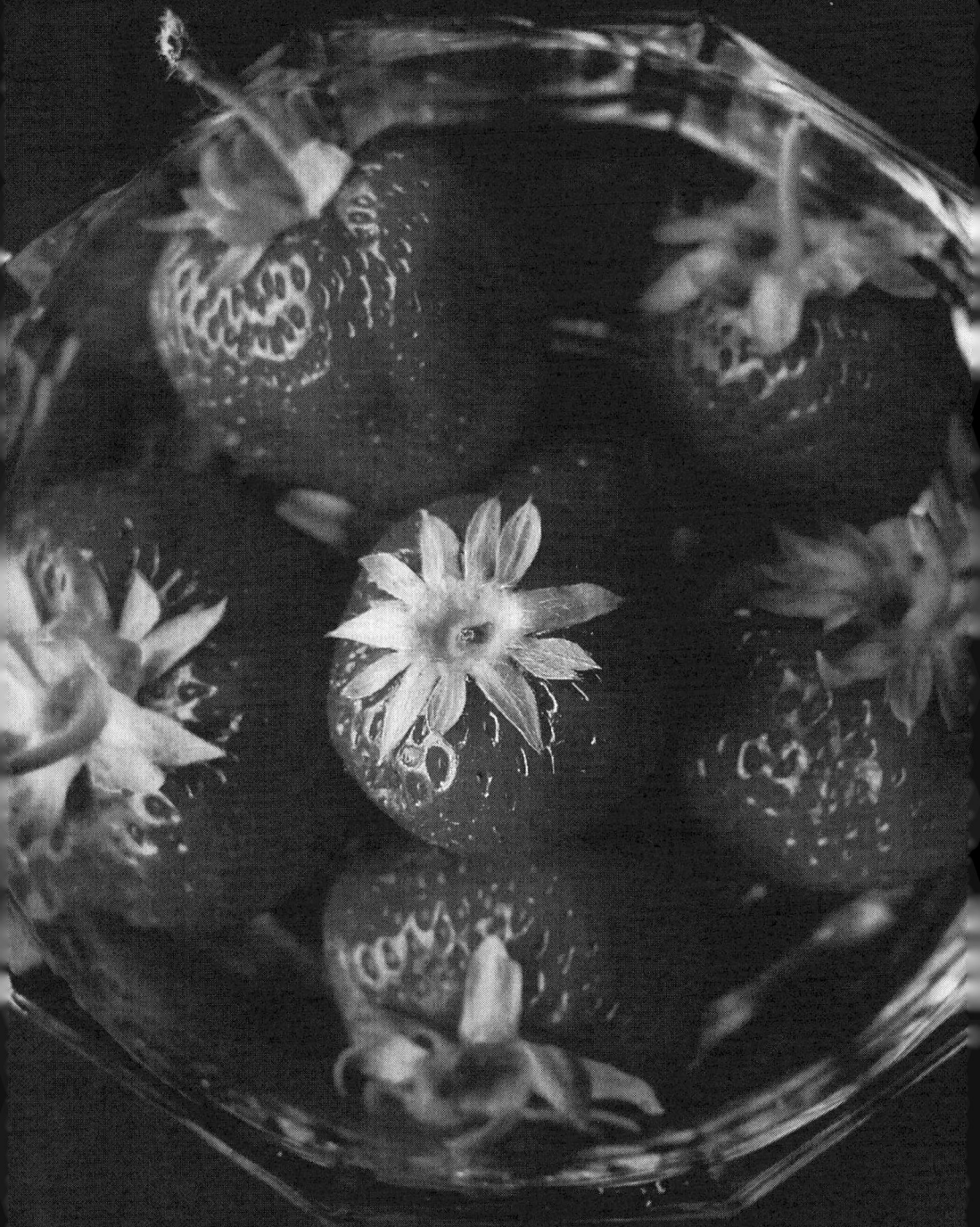

# The Ketogenic Diet

The first diet we will look at is the titular Ketogenic diet. This particular diet has been around for almost one hundred years, originating in the 1920's to help in several medical contexts. The most common use of the Keto diet in the early to mid twentieth century was to suppress epilepsy in children and adults alike.

Because fasting was the primary therapy, and relative "fix" for epilepsy at the time, the introduction of the Keto diet allowed for the patients to eat, which allowed them to maintain healthy weight and body mass, while reaping similar benefits of fasting in regards to their epileptic tendencies.

With the history and medical applications presented, one large question probably remains in your minds...

## Part 1: What Exactly is the Ketogenic Diet?

The Keto diet is a low-carb diet. It, like other similar low-carb diets, is designed around limiting one's intake of carbohydrates throughout a day or week to guide the body into burning fats. Because carbohydrates provide the body with proper "fuel" to burn throughout the day.

The "problem," if you want to call it that, comes into play with foods called "slow carbs." These foods include whole grains, legumes, nuts, seeds, and many types of beans and, like their name suggests, contain carbohydrates that burn slowly, over an extended period of time. While not intrinsically bad foods, the slow-burning carbohydrates give the body plenty of fuel to burn and plenty of time to burn it. If one were to eat too many of these slow-burning calories in a day, their body would never run out of fuel and, therefore, never burn the excess fat stored in the body.

The Keto diet limits the amount of slow-burning carbohydrates the body ingests in a given day or week so that the body has less new fuel to burn and can more quickly begin to burn the body's stored fats.

For those of you who have done your research regarding other types of diets may see a very stark similarity between the Keto diet and other low-carb diets out there. While it's true many low-carb diets work in similar manners to one another, the Keto diet adds an extra guideline to help burn off fat quicker and easier: Limits on proteins.

The Keto diet limits protein because of its ability to be converted into blood sugar (and fuel for the body). Limiting the protein in one's diet will increase the body's need to burn the excess body fat. While many other low-carb diets don't limit or restrict the intake of proteins into the body, often times those on other low-carb diets will begin to naturally drop the protein from their diets, which leads them to participating in the Keto diet accidently.

So, now that the basics concepts of the Keto diet are snuggly under your belt, you may wonder just how it all works out in your favor. The Keto diet revolves around the body creating and utilizing these molecules called ketones. These molecules are created from fat in the body for use as fuel if the body detects a lack of sugar in the blood stream. When one limits the carbohydrates and proteins from his or her diet, the body accesses its fat storage and creates its own fuel. Essentially, the body feels as though it's fasting (experiencing an extended amount of time without food intake) and works to prevent your body from running out of fuel. On the Keto diet, a person is almost tricking his or her body into burning fats directly by providing it with food, but not providing it with fuel.

In short, the Keto diet is a low-carb diet that relies on the limitation of carbohydrate and protein intake to force the body to burn fats rather than other "fuels" that it can get through the foods we eat everyday. This can lead to weight loss, a controllable hunger, and a steady stream of energy throughout the day (that means no more after lunch crashes!).

## Part 2: What Foods Can I/Can't I Eat?

As you may have guessed from the description of the Keto diet, carbohydrates and proteins are out of the question (in large or excessive quantities). Does that mean you have to stop eating them altogether? No, of course not, but remember, the amount of carbs and proteins you eat directly affects how much fuel you put into your body. The more fuel you put in, the less fat the body needs to burn.

So, what foods have a high amount of carbohydrates and proteins? The best advice anyone can give regardless of their choice of diet is, always check the label on the food. The serving size and nutritional information will save you hours of researching online.

Specifically, though, foods that should be avoided for their excess in carbohydrates are:

1. **Breads.** Yes, I hate to say it, but bread is a big supplier of carbohydrates. The worst part of bread being so high in carbs is that it's everywhere. From pizza and tacos, to gyros and breakfast sandwiches, it's hard to escape bread.

2. **Cereals.** Even the breakfast classic can have a downside. Cereals range from around 20 grams of carbs to roughly 30 per serving, so it's not a huge amount per bowl, but it is still something to be avoided. Not only do cereals contain a large amount of carbohydrates, but nearly 91 percent of their entire make up is carbohydrates. Yikes.

3. **Potatoes.** Potatoes are a versatile way to add mass to any meal, but they too come with a large amount of carbohydrates. While nowhere near as carb-dense as cereals are (potatoes only contain about 30 percent carbs), potatoes contain a larger amount of carbs throughout.

4. **Sodas. Pop. Coke. etc.** This one may seem like a give away, but avoid soda at all cost. Not only is it a source of excessive carbs, the sugars in the drink will mess with the sugars in your blood and throw your whole body through a loop (especially if you haven't drunk a soda in a while).

Those are only four examples of foods that should not be on your shopping list every single week. There are tons of other foods that have a less-than-desirable amount of carbs to watch out for. Always check the label before deciding to buy.

The second set of foods to avoid are those high in proteins. Unlike carbs, proteins play a large role in building muscles, so eating some on occasion (and in very limited amounts) will help your muscles stay the desired size.

1. Nuts. Every kind of nut has a high amount of either carbohydrates or protein (or both). They make for great slow-burning energy for longer

activities like hiking (which is why they're a main ingredient in trail mix), but on a day-to-day basis, that much protein would give the body too much to burn.

2. **Meats.** That's right, all meat has protein from beef, to pork, to chicken, to fish. While different kinds of meats have vastly different amounts of proteins in them, it's safe to say no meat should be eaten to excess.

But, wait, doesn't this book focus on using chicken in Ketogenic-based meals? While it's true that chicken is a meat and therefore has a relatively large amount of protein, it is also the best choice for consumption while on the Keto diet.

The purpose of this book is to introduce you, the reader, to the Keto diet. Not to convince you to become a vegetarian. Meat (or another source of protein, if you prefer) plays a large role in muscle development. While meat is something that shouldn't be eaten for every meal, there are a few guidelines to help you choose the right meat for the meals you do crave something with more protein.

Beef and pork both have higher amounts of protein, and higher fat content generally, than chicken does. While a hamburger can be the perfect summertime grill food, the excess protein and fats can leave the body with extra fuel and extra fat (meaning it not only is your body not burning the fat it has stored away already, but it's adding fat on top of it).

Fish is the lightest meat in terms of proteins and fat and can be a delicious and healthy meat. But, due to a variety of issues (including the possibility of mercury poisoning), fish should not be eaten in excess.

That really only leaves us with chicken. Chicken has moderate levels of protein and is typically a much leaner meat than beef or pork. While uncooked chicken can have a high-risk for disease, a chicken cooked all the way through does not share the same risks that fish does when eaten more often. Chicken, in essence, is the most versatile meat for our dietary needs.

Those are the plain and simple basics of the Keto diet and now you have two options. If this seems like the diet you want to stick to with no other information regarding the Paleo diet or other dieting tips, you can flip over to Chapter 4 to begin learning about a few diets that follow the Keto guidelines.

If, on the other hand, you want to learn a bit more about the Paleo diet and read a few tips to help you make the most of any diet, keep on reading.

# CHAPTER 2

# The Paleo Diet

This particular book mostly covers the basics of and recipes revolving around the Keto diet, but a lot of the recipes discovered and invented for people who are using the Keto diet tend to also be applicable to the Paleo diet as well.

For the sake of clarification as well as the sake of information, I've decided to include this chapter regarding the Paleo diet because, in all honesty, the diets are very similar to one another.

My dive into what makes the Paleo diet a worthwhile diet in its own right will be relatively short and less descriptive than the previous look into the basics of the Keto diet. The purpose of this chapter is to simply illustrate what makes the Paleo diet viable and how it is similar and different than the Keto diet.

## Part 1: What Exactly is the Paleo Diet?

The Paleolithic diet (or Paleo diet for short) focuses on foods that our ancestors would have eaten million of years ago. The central point of the Paleo diet is if our neanderthal ancestors could have had access to it, it's good for our bodies. There's a huge emphasis on restricting any and all processed foods from your diet as well as refined sugars and unhealthy fats.

## Part 2: What foods Can I/ Can't I Eat?

When abiding by the rules of the Paleo diet, like any diet, there are certain foods that you can eat, and there are certain foods to avoid. While the Keto diet tends to suggest certain aspects of food to avoid (carbohydrates and proteins), the Paleo diet focus on types of foods that aren't as beneficial for your body as others—Like the description of the Paleo diet says, the "good" foods are those that are naturally found in the world.

Foods that you can eat while on the Paleo diet:

1. **Fruits and vegetables.** Because of our collective hunter and gatherer past, fruits and vegetables are the perfect natural food to eat.

2. **Seafood and lean meat.** Where the Keto diet and Paleo diet cross is the meat section of your local grocery store. Both diets agree that seafood is alright to eat in small doses, as well as leaner meats such as chicken and other birds, while avoiding the fat-heavy meats such as beef and pork.

3. **Nuts.** The high protein in nuts help feed the body and give it natural energy. Nuts also include fats that the body can burn for energy.

Another area where the Paleo diet differs greatly from the Keto diet is the types of food to avoid. While the Keto diet suggests avoiding those foods high in carbohydrates and proteins, the Paleo diet strongly suggests avoiding a lot of foods that are common in an everyday diet because of their less than natural origins.

Foods that you should avoid while on the Paleo diet:

1. **Milk-based products.** Easily one of the hardest things to give up for those who are used eating them are milk-based products. This includes milk, cheese, yogurt, and plenty of other foods.

2. **Alcohols.** While any diet will tell you to avoid heavy use of alcohol (because, after all, a beer is just empty calories), the Paleo diet suggests that our bodies aren't designed to handle alcohol and, therefore, we shouldn't drink it.

3. **Processed foods and refined sugars.** Like alcohol, processed foods and refined sugars are often on many people's "avoid" list, but the Paleo diet pushes it further. Rather than limiting the amount of fats and sugars ingested, the Paleo diet's rules are pretty strict on restricting them from your diet entirely.

## Part 3: Similarities and Differences Between Diets

After reading about the Keto diet and the Paleo diet in the first two chapters of the book, the similarities and differences between the two may have become clear. Both diets revolve around the idea that our bodies are built specifically for eating a set palette of foods to maintain efficient health. While the Keto diet suggests that we need to avoid foods full of "fuels" for our bodies (such as those found in carbohydrates and proteins), the Paleo diet suggests that the only food we should put into our bodies are those found naturally on Earth.

Why are these two so different? The Paleo diet, in its focus on natural foods, doesn't necessarily mean that the diet has to be low carbohydrate like the Keto diet is. When someone is dedicated to the Paleo diet lifestyle, they usually exert more energy than other diets and need the excess energy to keep them healthy. What this means is carbohydrates *may* make up a reasonable amount of energy in someone's Paleo diet while that same person would avoid carbohydrates regardless of how they go about handling the Keto diet.

The amount of fat between the two diets can differ greatly. The Keto diet isn't absolutely against fat because it doesn't provide the body another source of fuel to burn. Rather, fat as it stands, is what the Keto diet is designed to burn. As long as the body doesn't have the body fuels found in carbs and proteins, it will still burn fat regardless of source.

The Paleo diet also allows fat, but for different reasons. The fat provides extra fuel on top of the carbs to help extend your active time. The Paleo diet doesn't necessarily mean that every person has to eat foods with a high fat content, but fat works with longer burning fuels so many people abiding by the Paleo lifestyle tend to eat some higher fat foods.

The biggest and arguably most noticeable difference is the allowance of milk and other dairy-based foods. Nature dictates that most mammals actually become lactose intolerant as they age to allow younger siblings to benefit from their mother's milk. Because of this, our ancestors wouldn't have drunk milk (especially milk from another species like cows) or wouldn't have eaten milk-based foods.

On the other hand, if you are more inclined to follow the rules of the Keto diet, milk is an easy way to augment your fat intake so you don't have to eat protein-dense meats or nuts to get that fat.

The Keto diet and the Paleo diet are similar in a lot of aspects, but differ in a few major areas. Both diets have many, many, many different variations, some of which have very few differentiating variables between them. Because of the large amount of variations of diets, there are many types of Keto diets that almost cross into Paleo territory and vice versa. If you break away from your Keto rules and cross into Paleo rules, it's alright because of the vast amount of similarities that accompany all of the differences.

# Healthy Diet Tips

*W*hile the Keto diet may seem like a relatively simple set of rules to follow to help you lose weight, it can be difficult to abide by the diet's guidelines (food temptation is everywhere, after all).

The following tips are designed and organized to help you not only make the most of your experience with the Keto diet, but are also here to help you find strategies to keep you on the right track, even when that pizza is tempting you. The tips chosen for this section range from obvious to some, to unique and generally unheard of. With that, a few of the tips are applicable to many other diets, but work astoundingly well with the Keto diet in particular.

### Tip 1: Get up and move

One thing that will keep your body's metabolism up and your fat burning continuous is to simply get up and move around. If you have a desk job, or if you're a student and dedicate a lot of time to homework, find times to take breaks throughout the day. Even a simple walk up and down the hallway will help.

### Tip 2: Sleep well and consistently

I understand that sleeping through the night may not always be up to you as stress and other internal and external variables may drag your from under your covers. But sleeping through the night consistently will allow your body to work at peak efficiency.

It also helps to keep a strict sleep schedule, so maybe staying out until 2 AM on both Friday night and Saturday night may not be the best idea if you have to work at 8 AM on Monday.

### Tip 3: Stick to a schedule

Keeping a sleep schedule is important, but keeping a schedule of your everyday will help your body get into the groove of a new diet. Setting aside time to eat (and setting aside exactly what you will eat for each meal) is a great way to avoid excess snacking and uncontrollable hunger.

Keeping a schedule will also help you get in your daily exercise as well.

### Tip 4: Drink water

Drinking water is easily the most obvious health tip, but it's also easily one of the most ignored health tips out there. Keep a water bottle with you and drink it throughout the day. The last thing you want is for your body to become dehydrated, especially when exercising or dieting.

### Tip 5: Find your mental and emotional balance

While it's easier said than done for a lot of people, finding your mental and emotional balance is an important aspect of any and all healthy lifestyle. There are a large number of ways to help you achieve your personal mental and emotional balance, and many of these ways may work for you personally and not others. Avoid stress by planning ahead, sleep well, take time out of your day to meditate, and other activities can help reduce mental and emotional burnout and keep your body and mind healthy and balanced.

# CHAPTER 4

# Ketogenic-Centric Recipes

*B*ecause the Keto diet suggests a limited amount of carbs and proteins, it only makes sense that recipes designed to work with the diet focus on good foods with as little carbs and proteins as possible.

While a great way to avoid both of these nutrients is to avoid meat (chicken included), your body does need a bit of protein to build muscle and keep you strong. With that in mind, the following recipes follow the Keto diet's guidelines, while introducing chicken to give you the limited amount of protein your body needs (and let's be honest, while fruits and vegetables are delicious, a nice piece of meat adds variety and flavor to your daily diet).

# Keto Meal #1:
# Keto Coconut Pancakes

Time used to prepare ingredients: 10 minutes
Time used to cook or bake ingredients: 3 minutes per pancakes
Total time to make this recipe: 25 minutes
(this can change depending on the size of your pancakes)

This recipe yields: four medium sized pancakes

## Ingredients:

- 1/4 cup (2 ounces) of vanilla almond milk
- 1 Tablespoon (1/2 of an ounce) of vanilla yogurt
- 3 Tablespoons (1 1/2 ounces) of Coconut flour
- 1 Tablespoon (1/2 of an ounce) sugar (natural is better)
- 3 egg whites
- 1/2 teaspoon (2 milliliters) imitation vanilla extract (you may use actual extract, but imitation works just as well because of the vanilla yogurt and vanilla almond milk).
- A pinch of coarse salt
- A pinch of baking powder

## Directions:

1.  Pull out your medium to medium large mixing bowl and throw in your coconut flour, sugar, coarse salt, and baking powder. Mix the ingredients well to combine them completely.

    a.  If you're worried about nonuniform texture in your mixture, you can sift the ingredients before hand, or use an electric mixture to make sure the ingredients fully combine.

2.  Set your dry mixture aside and pull out another mixing bowl (this one can be medium small). Separate the yolk and whites from your eggs and get rid of the egg yolks (you can set them aside for another recipe, or

throw them away. Most of the protein is in the egg's yolk, so use them wisely).

3. In your medium small mixing bowl, pour your imitation vanilla extract and egg whites and whisk them together until fluffy and consistent. The fluffier your egg whites are, the fluffier your pancakes will be!

4. Once your egg whites are your desired consistency, use a spatula to scrape the fluff onto the dry ingredients one scoop at a time. As you add the fluff to your dry ingredients, fold the mixture together gently. After you've mixed half of your egg whites in with your dry ingredients, add your vanilla yogurt and continue to fold your ingredients together.

5. Once the ingredients are folded together, add your vanilla almond milk and mix it into the other ingredients until a nice pancake batter has formed.

   a. It's important you don't stir too quickly or hard because it can damage the batter's texture.

6. Pull out a pan or skillet and set it on the stove top. Set the heat to low or medium low and wait for several minutes until the pan has completely heated up.

   a. To check your pan's heat, place your hand under running water and, while it's still wet, flick water droplets onto the pan. If the water moves around and evaporates, your pan is ready for your pancakes.

7. Once your pan is at the desired temperature, pour batter into the bottom and let cook for a few minutes. Once bubbles start to form in the center of your pancake (and the edges are golden brown), flip the pancake and let cook on the other side for two minutes or so.

8. Cook all of your pancakes one at a time (be patient) and stack on a plate to cool.

▸ If you don't have non-stick pans or skillets, use non-stick spray (or butter if you want to treat yourself) to prevent the pancakes from sticking to the surface.

▸ You can change the flavor of yogurt to alter the flavor of the pancakes (this goes for the milk as well).

▸ Because the recipe calls for a lot of vanilla ingredients, these pancakes go well with more vanilla yogurt as a side or other, fruit flavors such as strawberries, blueberries, and, if you're adventurous, pineapple.

# Keto Meal #2:
# The Keto Monte Cristo

Time used to prepare ingredients: less than 5 minutes
Time used to cook or bake ingredients: 3 minutes
Total time to make this recipe: around 10 minutes

This recipe yields: 1 sandwich

## Ingredients:

- 1/4 of a pound (4 ounces) of sliced ham (about 2 medium thin slices)
- 1/4 of a pound (4 ounces) of sliced turkey (about 2 medium thin slices)
- 1 cup (8 ounces) shredded cheddar cheese (two slices also work)
- 3 low carb or gluten free pancakes (follow recipe on box or use the pancakes we made in recipe 1)

## Directions:

1. Start off by making your low carb or gluten free pancakes. If you are using powdered mix (which is totally alright!), follow the direction on the box. Chances are it will have you mix the powder with water then pour the wet mixture into your pan or skillet and turn over once bubbles start to form in the center.

   a. If you are brave enough to attempt to make your own (they are pretty easy) then follow the directions for the low carb pancakes in recipe 1.

2. Keep the stove on after your pancakes are finished, you will use it to properly heat your meat to give it a nice texture. Turn the stove top to low so as not to burn the meat.

3.  Place 1 slice of ham into the pan or skillet and immediately add one fourth of your shredded cheddar cheese directly onto the meat, being extra careful to not let any fall directly onto the metal of the pan (as cheese can burn easily).

4.  Now, do the same thing with your turkey. Take your slice and add it to the pan. Sprinkle another fourth of your cheddar cheese on top of the turkey.

5.  Cover the pan or skillet with a lid (it doesn't need to be tight fitting) and let cook for one minute or until the cheese is nice and melted.

6.  Add one of your three pancakes back to the pan or skillet and sprinkle one half of the remaining cheddar cheese to the top. Once the cheese begins to melt (it doesn't have to fully melt) place your ham and cheese directly on top.

7.  Then, add your second pancake and sprinkle the remaining cheddar cheese. Quickly, place the turkey and cheese on top.

8.  Finally, add your last pancake to the stack and press down on your tower to press all of it together. Move your meal to a plate and chow down!

Extra tips for this recipe:

⇒ If you want to add a bit of flavor, there are a few ways to do so:
   ⇒ Maple syrup is a tasty, if not sugary treat that many people enjoy.
   ⇒ Balsamic Vinegar of your choosing can add a bit of tartness.
   ⇒ If you really want to get crazy, you can dip your sandwich into tomato soup or bisque.

# Keto Meal #3:
# Low Carb Breakfast Chicken Sausage

*Time used to prepare ingredients:* 15 minutes
*Time used to cook or bake ingredients:* 10 minutes
*Total time to make this recipe:* 25 minutes

*This recipes yields:* 8 Patties (enough for 4 people)

## Ingredients:

- 3/4 teaspoon (3 milliliters) parsley
- 1/2 teaspoon (2 milliliters) garlic powder
- 1/2 teaspoon (2 milliliters) onion powder
- 1/4 teaspoon (1 milliliter) thyme
- 1/8 teaspoon (1/2 milliliter) freshly ground nutmeg
  - (pre-ground nutmeg works, too, but nothing beats the fresh flavors of freshly ground)
- 1/8 teaspoon (1/2 milliliter) red pepper flakes
- 1 teaspoon (5 milliliters) sage
- 1 pound (16 ounces) of ground chicken
- 1 pinch of ground cloves
- Pepper and salt to taste
  - Usually, the recipe doesn't require more salt, but pepper will always make the sausage pop.

## Directions:

1. Pull out your largest mixing bowl and throw your ground chicken meat into it. Be sure to drain excess fat from the packaging before putting the chicken in the mixing bowl to avoid adding extra fat or meat juice to your recipe. Mix the ground chicken a bit so that it separates (you don't want a block of meat in your bowl).

**18**

2. Toss your onion powder, garlic powder, pepper, red pepper flakes, sage, thyme, nutmeg, sage, and ground cloves into your mixing bowl with the ground chicken and mix. You want to mix until all of the herbs and spices are equally spread throughout the chicken (avoid clumps at all costs!).

3. Once the herbs and spices are well spread throughout the chicken, use your hands to create small patties out of the seasoned meat (around half the size of a hockey puck). You could use a dry measuring cup coated with nonstick spray to help you get the meat into even servings, but scooping the meat by hand is much easier and efficient.

4. Pull out a large pan or skillet and place it on your stove top. Set the heat to medium (or medium hot if you like a bit of crisp around the edges). Coat the pan in a nonstick butter, margarine, oil, or spray (do this especially if you are not using a nonstick pan).

   a. While margarine and especially butter will add a nice fatty flavor to your sausage, oil will allow for the same nonstick applications without the excess fat. You can also use flavored olive oils to get a unique blend of flavors.

5. To check the pan or skillet's heat, flick water onto it. If the water bounces and evaporates, you can pour in your oil and add your sausage (do this BEFORE adding the oil). Once the pan reaches the desired temperature, place your formed patties into the pan. Place them in one at a time to avoid splashing and make sure the patties don't overlap too much.

6. Cook for roughly a minute and a half one side (until the bottom is nice and brown with a bit of crispiness) then flip each patty (one at a time) to cook for another minute on the other side.

7. Serve your chicken sausage with syrup or alongside eggs or pancakes and enjoy!

## Extra tips for this recipe:

➡ Be creative with your sausage. Try replacing one fourth of the chicken with finely diced apples for a unique flavor experience.

➡ Don't shy away from changing up the herbs and spices and their amounts. If you don't like cloves, for example, don't add them and add more onion.

➡ Chicken sausage works well with anything from fruits and vegetables to other meats or heavy breads (although large amounts of breads should be avoided).

# Keto Meal #4: Low Carb, Low Calorie Chicken Salad

Time used to prepare ingredients: 10 minutes
Time used to cook or bake ingredients: 0 minutes
Total time to make this recipe: 10 minutes

This recipe yields: 1 1/2 cup of salad (about 3 serving)

## Ingredients:

- 1/3 pound (roughly 5 ounces) of chicken
  - You can use ground chicken or you can mince full breasts if you really want to make this recipe from scratch.
- 1 large egg
- 1 stick of celery
- 1/2 Tablespoon (1/4 of an ounce) dill pickle relish
- 1/3 cup (2 1/2 ounces) of Mayonnaise
- 1 teaspoon (5 milliliters) dijon mustard
- 2 Tablespoons (10 milliliters) parsley
- 1 green onion
- 1/2 clove of garlic
- Pepper and salt to taste

## Directions:

1. Set your stove's heat to medium or medium high and place a medium sized pan or skillet over the flame. Cook your chicken until golden brown. If you decided to purchase whole chicken breasts, you'll need cut the cooked chicken into small cubes or strands (the finer the better). Set the cooked and drained chicken aside.

2. Finely chop your celery, green onion, and parsley. Like the chicken, the finer the cut, the better texture and consistency your salad will have. A food processor is also a completely acceptable method of cutting these ingredients. Just throw the celery, green onion, and parsley in together and pulse until fine.

3. Mix your celery, green onion, and parsley in a large mixing bowl and slowly add your fine cuts of chicken.

4. On the stove top, place a large pot with cold water and add some salt. Drop in your one large egg and add more water so that the surface is about an inch above the top of the egg. Turn the stove to medium heat and bring to a boil. Once the water is boiling, cover the pot with a tight fitting lid and set aside for the egg to finish cooking.

5. Set the egg in the refrigerator for at least three hours to allow it to cool and solidify. Once it's cooled down, cut the egg (yolk and whites) into fine pieces (Again, the finer the better). Add the egg to your mixing bowl with your celery, green onion, parsley, and chicken mixture and stir until combined.

6. Measure out your dijon mustard, minced garlic, dill pickle relish, mayonnaise, and pepper and salt and turn the mixture until well combined.

   a. Turning the mixture, rather than stirring it, will keep the ingredients' from getting smashed and keep their textures separate (a variety of textures will feel better to eat than a pile of mush).

7. Serve on bread or with greens, or just eat it with a fork!

🔆 Extra tips for this recipe:

⇢ Hot sauce and chicken always go well together. Add some spice to make a buffalo chicken salad!

⇢ You can leave out most ingredients if you don't like the flavor or texture, or simply don't want the additional calories. The hard boiled egg, for example, can be left out completely to make the chicken salad even healthier and less protein dense.

⇢ In a vegetarian mood? Switch of the chicken for tofu!

# Keto Meal #5: Chicken With Walnuts and Fennel Salad

Time used to prepare ingredients: 5 minutes
Time used to cook or bake ingredients: 10 minutes
Total time to make this recipe: 15 minutes

This recipe yields: 1 large salad or 6 individual sized salads

## Ingredients:

- 1/4 cup (2 ounces) of toasted walnuts
- 1 1/2 cups (12 ounces) of fennel
- 1/2 pound (8 ounces) of skinless and boneless chicken breasts
- 2 Tablespoons (1 ounce) fennel fronds
- 2 Tablespoons(1 ounce) juice from a lemon
- 1/4 cup (2 ounces) of mayonnaise
- 2 Cloves of garlic
- 1/8 teaspoon (1/2 milliliter) of cayenne
- 2 Tablespoons (10 milliliters) walnut oil
- Pepper and salt to preference

## Directions:

1. The first step is to cook your chicken. Place a medium to a medium large pan or skillet on your stove top. Set the heat to medium and let the pan or skillet heat up for a few minutes. Flick water onto the bottom to test the heat.

2. Place your chicken breasts onto the heated pan and cook for roughly 3 minutes until the bottom is brown. Flip the chicken over and cook for an additional 3 minutes until the chicken is fully cooked through.

a. If you aren't using a non-stick pan, be sure to spray the bottom with non-stick spray or use olive oil to prevent sticking. These are acceptable if you are using a non-stick pan, also, and want to make sure no sticking occurs.

3. Once the chicken is fully cooked (it's important to cook the chicken fully), take it from the pan and cut it into cubes or strips (it's up to you).

4. Pull out a large mixing bowl and place in your fully cooked chicken. Chop both the fennel and walnuts and toss them over the chicken. Mix the ingredients until they are well combined.

5. In a separate mixing bowl, throw together the mayonnaise, fennel fronds, cayenne, lemon juice, and walnut oil. Stir the ingredients until fully combined and smooth. This is your dressing for your salad.

6. Pour your newly mixed dressing over your chicken, fennel, and walnut mixture and toss everything together.

7. Cover the mixing bowl with cling wrap or tinfoil and throw it into the refrigerator for at least an hour. If you have the time, leave the mixture covered and in the refrigerator for 3 to 4 hours because the longer you keep it covered, the more the flavors will fuse together.

8. Pull the salad out and serve over fresh greens like spinach or lettuce.

Extra tips for this recipe:

➡ The walnuts can be switched out for another nut, so try using your favorites when you make the recipe.

➡ If you want more citrus in your salad, add some cranberries with your walnuts.

# Keto Meal #6:
# Keto Thin Crust Pizza

Time used to prepare ingredients: 30 minutes
Time used to cook or bake ingredients: 1 hour and 30 minutes
Total time to make this recipe: 2 hours

This recipe yields: 1 pizza (6 servings)

## Ingredients:

- 1 cup (8 ounces) of chia seeds
- 1 stalk of cauliflower
- 1/2 bag of cauliflower florets work just as well (yes, even if frozen).
- 1 cup (8 ounces) water
- 1 teaspoon (5 milliliters) salt
- 1/2 cup (4 ounces) of heavy cream
- 1/2 cup (4 ounces) of cream cheese
- 1/2 cup (4 ounces) of parmesan cheese
- 3 Tablespoons (1/2 ounce) of olive oil
- 2 cloves of garlic
- Pepper and salt

## Directions:

1. Turn the heat on your oven up to 100 degrees fahrenheit.

2. Cut the cauliflower into small pieces and throw them into your food processor. Chop the cauliflower into a fine consistency (you don't have to use a food processor, but the finer and more consistent the cauliflower, the better. A food processor makes it much easier to do).

3. Pour the chia seeds into an herb grinder and grind the seeds into a fine powder (this will replace the flour for the crust, so make sure the seeds are ground very fine).

4.  Pull out a medium mixing bowl and throw together your finely chopped cauliflower and ground chia seeds. Mix the two together until combined.

5.  Pour the water, olive oil, and a bit of salt into the mixture and combine again. It takes a few minutes, but you want to make sure there are no clumps in your dough.

6.  Cover with a towel or rag (or a damp paper towel) and set aside for 15 to 20 minutes.

7.  Take out a cookie sheet and coat it with non-stick spray or olive oil (olive oil can add a nice flavor that non-stick spray can't).

8.  Once the dough is done sitting, place it on the cookie sheet and spread it so it covers all of the bottom (the dough will stretch and stay if you keep pulling it).

    a.  If you want, you can adjust how thick your crust is. Using a smaller pan will make a thicker crust (which requires more baking), and using a large sheet or multiple sheets will yield thinner crusts.

9.  Place your cookie sheet(s) on the center rack of your pre-heated oven and let bake for 50 to 70 minutes (time will vary based on how thick or thin your crust is). Once the crust is fully baked and dry, pull it from the heat and turn the oven to 400 degrees fahrenheit.

10. Pull out your food processor again and toss in you parmesan, heavy cream, cream cheese, and garlic (be sure to peel the garlic first). Pulse the mixture until a paste has formed.

11. Spread your sauce over the top of the crust and place into your pre-heated oven for 10 minutes more.

12. Once the crust is nice and brown, pull from the heat and cut into 6 slices. Serve and enjoy!

## Extra tips for this recipe:

➠ While the sauce has enough flavor, some people may want to add more texture to their pizza. Feel free to add sliced tomatoes, olives, pineapples, peppers, or other toppings to your pizza to personalize it.

# Paleo-Centric Recipes

The largest difference between the Keto diet and the Paleo diet is the focus on where daily calories come from. While the Keto diet suggests that carbs and proteins be generally avoided (or at least limited in one's daily diet), the Paleo diet suggests that the calories can come from any foods that you can find naturally on Earth.

The following recipes focus on using foods naturally found on Earth, which require no processing before arriving to your local grocery store. Many of these recipes can be included with the Keto diet, but are in this section because of the focus on natural and unprocessed foods.

# Paleo Meal #1: Baked Eggs Flavored with Italian Herbs

Time used to prepare ingredients: 20 minutes
Time used to cook or bake ingredients: 15 minutes
Total time to make this recipe: 35 minutes

## Ingredients:

- 6 eggs (both the yolks and the whites)
- 1 Tablespoon (1/2 ounce) of shredded parmesan cheese
- 1/8 cup (1 ounce) of heavy cream
- 1 Tablespoon (1/2 ounce) of unsalted butter
- 1 garlic clove
- 1 teaspoon (5 milliliters) thyme
- 1 teaspoon (5 milliliters) parsley
- 1 teaspoon (5 milliliters) oregano
- Pepper and salt

## Directions:

1. Crank the heat on your oven to 350 degrees fahrenheit. Make sure your oven rack is in the center position. Too low and your eggs won't cook evenly, too high and your eggs may cook too quickly on top.

2. Mince the clove of garlic, and finely chop your thyme, parsley, and oregano. In a small bowl (it can even be a dinner bowl), mix your herbs and shredded parmesan cheese. Set the bowl aside and forget about it for a few minutes.

3. In a large bowl (or oven dish), pour your heavy cream and butter. If your butter is not melted yet, don't worry, just place the solid butter in the dish with the cream.

4. Set the cream and butter into the oven and let heat for five minutes (just so the mutter melts and the heavy cream is warm).

   a. If you so desire, you may heat the heavy cream and butter in a microwave safe dish then transfer it to the oven dish.

5. Crack your eggs into a large bowl while your heavy cream and butter heat up. From here, you can do one of two things:

   a. You can whisk the eggs—like you would do to scrambled eggs.

   b. You can keep the yolks intact.

6. Regardless of if you keep the yolks intact or not, remove the now warm heavy cream and butter from the oven (or microwave) and pour the eggs over them. If you decided to whisk the egg whites and yolks together, you may want to give the whole mixture a quick stir.

7. Sprinkle your herb and cheese mixture over the top of your eggs. To add flavor, grind and sprinkle pepper and salt to your liking.

8. Toss your oven dish back into the oven and set the timer to 15 minutes. Once the timer goes off, press the eggs down with the tongs of a fork to see if the eggs are cooked thoroughly (if there's some wiggle, place the mixture back into the oven for an additional three minutes).

9. Once the eggs are ready, remove them from the oven and set the entire oven dish onto your stovetop or cooling rack for one minute. Once the minutes is up, cut and serve!

## Extra tips for this recipe:

➡ It's true that eggs aren't technically chickens yet, but for the sake of breakfast tradition, eggs work well to provide you the protein you need throughout the day. If you feel as though you need more protein on a daily basis, it is best to eat it in the morning to allow your body more physical time to absorb it.

➡ These eggs work well for sandwiches, as side dishes, or the main course of any breakfast or brunch.

➡ Do you want to eat eggs, but want to avoid the protein? Separate your yolks and egg whites and cook for ten minutes at 350 degrees fahrenheit instead.

# Paleo Meal #2: Stuffed Paleo Avocados

Time used to prepare ingredients: 10 minutes
Time used to cook or bake ingredients: 0 minutes
Total time to make this recipe: 10 minutes

This recipes yields: 2 Avocados (2 serving)

## Ingredients:

- 2 Avocado
- 2 bunch of chives
- 2 tins of sardines
- 2 Tablespoon (1 ounce) of lemon juice
- 2 Tablespoon (1 ounce) mayonnaise
- 1/2 teaspoon (2 milliliters) turmeric
- Pepper and salt

## Directions:

1. Cut each of the avocados in half and remove the pit. Drain the sardines in your sink. Either chop the sardines into small pieces or use a food processor to cut them into small piece. set them aside for the time being.

2. Using a spoon, or small ice cream scoop, scoop out the center of the avocados to make a bowl (you want to make sure you leave plenty of avocado to eat).

3. In a medium-sized mixing bowl, place your chopped sardines, ground turmeric, mayonnaise, and chives. Mix your ingredients until they are all well combined.

4. Take the extra scoops of your avocados and throw them into the mixing bowl with your sardines and other ingredients. Use a fork to mash the

avocado into the texture you like (some people like it smooth, others like it with chunks of avocado; it's up to you).

5.  Once the avocado is to your liking, either squeeze or pour the lemon juice over it and fold it gently into the mixture.

6.  Scoop the mixture back into your avocado bowls and add pepper and salt to taste.

## ⚡ Extra tips for this recipe:

➡ Sardines aren't everyone's favorite. If you don't like the small fish, feel free to leave them out and replace them with another form of protein (chicken works exceptionally well).

➡ Want a spicier avocado? Add cayenne on top to give it extra heat!

➡ This recipe doubles as a fairly unique guacamole recipe. Instead of making avocado bowls, scoop all of the avocados into the bowl and serve with chips!

# Paleo Meal #3:
# Sausage and Egg Breakfast or Lunch Casserole

Time used to prepare ingredients: 30 minutes
Time used to cook or bake ingredients: 40 minutes to 60 minutes
Total time to make this recipe: 1 hour 1o minutes to 1 hour and 30 minutes

This recipe yields: 1 casserole (4 servings)

## Ingredients:

- Your favorite brand of pie crust
- 2 large eggs
- 3 slices of bacon (the thicker, the better)
- 1/2 pound (8 ounces) of ground sausage (chicken sausage works really well!)
- 1/4 cup (2 ounces) of cream cheese
- 1 cloves of garlic
- 1/2 red onion
- 1/8 cup (1 ounce) of chives
- 1/2 cup (4 ounces) of shredded cheddar cheese
- Olive oil
- Pepper and salt

## Directions:

1. Make the pie crust you chose to use (follow the directions on the box). Preheat the oven in accordance with the instruction on the pie crust of your choice.

2. Get out your pie pan (or 9x9 oven safe dish) and spread the pie crust over it. Place another, smaller bowl on top of your pie crust so that it stays as flat as possible and place it in your oven's center rack for around 15 minutes.

3. Peel the garlic and mince it, throw it into a non-stick pan with some olive oil. Turn the heat to medium and let the smell of garlic fill your kitchen.

4. While the garlic is heating up in the olive oil, peel your red onion and chop it. Once you can smell the garlic, throw the onion into the pan or skillet with them and stir a few times to coat with olive oil. While that cooks, cut your bacon into quarter inch pieces.

5. Once the red onion begins to sweat, toss the chopped bacon into the pan or skillet and stir everything together. Let the mixture sit until the bacon is nice and crispy (about 4 minutes).

6. While the bacon cooks, take the ground sausage and add it to the same pan as the garlic, red onion, and bacon. Cook until the sausage is browned (about 6 minutes) and set to the side.

7. Preheat your oven to 400 degrees fahrenheit.

8. Pull out a medium to medium large mixing bowl and crack both of the eggs into it. Whisk the eggs together until smooth, then add the cream cheese, pepper, and salt. Again, whisk the eggs until everything is well combined.

9. Once the cream cheese in combined with the eggs, pour in the shredded cheddar cheese and whisk again.

10. Finally, dump the chives into the egg mixture and whisk one more time.

11. Pull your crust out again and spread your bacon and sausage mixture into it. Make sure all of the meat and onions are evenly spread throughout the crust.

12. Slowly, pour the egg mixture over the bacon and sausage in the crust (too fast and the egg will splash).

13. Toss the pie back into the oven and bake for another 25 minutes.

14. Once the buzzer goes off, take the pie from the heat and set aside for 10 minutes to let cool.

15. Slice and serve!

## ☀ Extra tips for this recipe:

➠ While this recipe is an egg-based casserole (a common breakfast food) you can make it for any meal.

➠ If you don't want sausage in the middle of the day, feel free to replace it with another protein. Chicken, pork, and even tofu work as perfect substitutes.

➠ A large number of sauces work well with this casserole: Hot sauce, hollandaise, and even a nice mango salsa can add a wide variety of flavors to this dish.

# Paleo Meal #4: Paleo Buffalo Chicken

Time used to prepare ingredients: 45 minutes
Time used to cook or bake ingredients: 20 minutes
Total time to make this recipe: 1 hour 5 minutes

This recipe yields: 4 - 6 servings
(depending on the size of the chicken breasts you use)

## Ingredients:

- 2 Tablespoons (1 ounce) Oregano
- 1 1/2 Tablespoons (3/4 ounce) Garlic powder
- 1 1/2 Tablespoons (3/4 ounce) Ground cumin
- 2 Tablespoons (1 ounce) Chili powder
- 3 teaspoons (1/2 ounce) of Cayenne pepper
- 1/2 cup (4 ounces) of water
- 1/2 cup (4 ounces) of cider vinegar
- 2 pounds (32 ounces) of boneless and skinless chicken breasts

## Directions:

1. The first thing to do is to prepare the chicken. First, cut each chicken breast into long strips (you can get between 3 and 5 strips from each chicken breast).

2. Pull out a large ziplock bag and place the chicken in it with the cider vinegar, cayenne pepper, and water.

3. Shake your chicken and other ingredients so that the chicken becomes completely covered. If you need to, place the bag on a surface and use your fingers to push the chicken around from the outside to cover it all.

4. Place the bag in the refrigerator for 30 to 45 minutes.

35

5. Turn the heat on your oven to 350 degrees fahrenheit and pull out a large baking sheet.

6. Pull your chicken bag from the refrigerator and place the chicken strips onto the baking sheet.

7. In a medium sized mixing bowl, mix the oregano, chili powder, garlic powder, and cumin so that they are evenly combined.

8. Sprinkle your mixture of herbs and spices onto one side of your chicken, then turn each strip over and sprinkle the other side.

9. Place your seasoned chicken strips on the oven's center rack and bake for 18 to 23 minutes (check after 18 minutes to check for doneness).

## Extra tips for this recipe:

➥ If the herb and spices don't quite meet your flavor standards, try altering the amounts in small amounts, or removing certain herbs altogether.

➥ Try a variety of dipping sauces to add even more flavor to your chicken strips (they also taste great on their own!).

# Pressure Cooker Recipes

*O*ur third and final set of recipes revolve around a kitchen appliance that many people tend to overlook: The pressure cooker. The pressure cooker is the ideal "set it and forget it" tool to use when making a large variety of foods. The pressure cooker is the best unless you want to wait half a day for your food to be cooked (like with the more common slow cooker or crock pot).

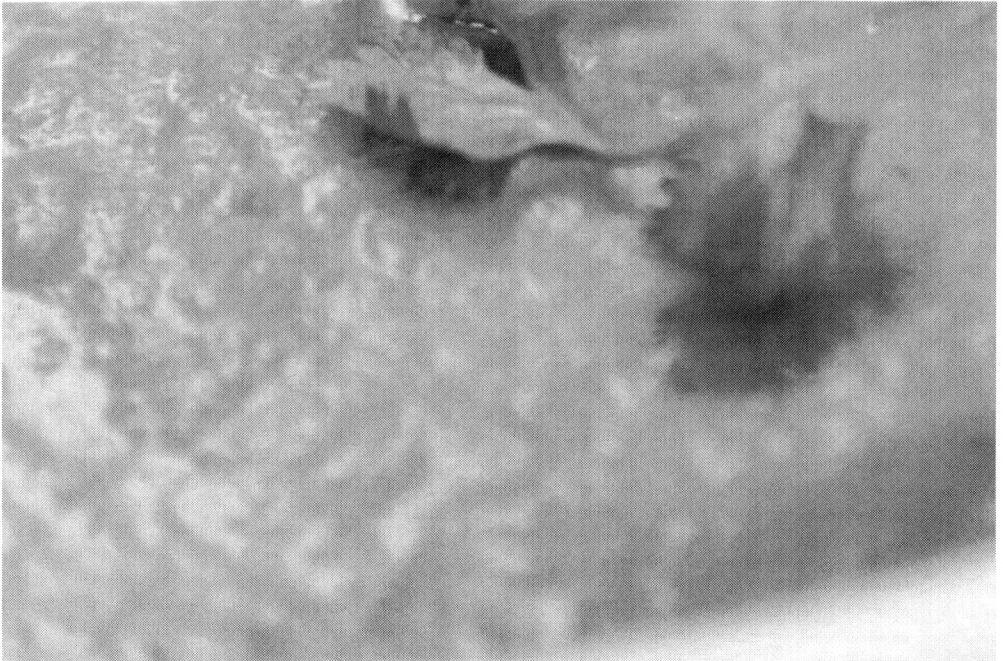

# Pressure Cooker Meal #1: Low Carb Spicy Chicken Soup

Time used to prepare ingredients: 10 minutes
Time used to cook or bake ingredients: 10 minutes
Total time to make this recipe: 20 minutes

This recipe yields: 1 bowls of soup (1 servings)

## Ingredients:

➡ 1/2 cup (4 ounces) of chicken broth
➡ 1 Skinless and boneless chicken breast (1/2 pound or 8 ounces)
➡ 1/2 Tablespoon (1/2 ounce) powdered ranch dressing mix
➡ 1/8 cup (1 ounce) onion (roughly 1/4 of an onion)
➡ 1/4 cup (2 ounces) of celery (roughly 1 stalk)
➡ 1 Clove of garlic
➡ 1/3 cup (2 1/2 ounces) of hot sauce
➡ 1/2 cup (4 ounces) of heavy cream
➡ 1 cup (8 ounces) of shredded cheddar cheese

## Directions:

1.  Chop your celery and onion into chunks of your choosing. The common preference is about 1/4 to 1/2 an inch across for best texture and even cooking. Next, peel and mince the garlic.

2.  Pull out your pressure cooker and throw in your chopped vegetables, garlic, chicken, chicken broth, powdered ranch dressing mix, and hot sauce (everything except the heavy cream and shredded cheddar cheese).

3.  Cook your mixture in your pressure cooker for 10 minutes (you may need to wait until 14 minutes pass to make sure everything is cooked thoroughly).

4. Using tongs or two forks, remove the now fully cooked chicken from your pressure cooker and place onto a cutting board or large plate. Using two forks, pull the chicken apart to make thin strips of pulled meat. Return the pulled chicken to your pressure cooker.

5. Pour in the heavy cream and give the mixture a stir. Then, in 1/4 of a cup increments, pour in the shredded cheddar cheese, stirring constantly.

6. Use a ladle to spoon the soup into a bowl and serve either by itself or with chips or bread.

## Extra tips for this recipe:

➡ Hot sauce can make all the differences; try experimenting with different brands and bases of hot sauces to find a flavor that's perfect for you.

➡ Sour cream always works as a topping or side, as well as extra cheese, chips, and bread. While these sides may add a nice texture to your meal, they also add calories and carbs, so be careful how much you add.

# Pressure Cooker Meal #2: Quick and Easy Garlic Lemon Chicken

*Time used to prepare ingredients:* 10 minutes
*Time used to cook or bake ingredients:* 20 minutes
*Total time to make this recipe:* 30 minutes

*This recipe yields:* 3 - 4 servings of chicken

## Ingredients:

- 2 pounds (32 ounces) of skinless and boneless chicken breasts
- 1 onion
- 5 cloves of garlic
- 1/2 cup (4 ounces) of chicken broth
- 1 Tablespoon (1/2 ounce) of lard
- 1 teaspoon (5 milliliters) of parsley
- 1/4 teaspoon (1 milliliter) paprika
- 1/4 cup (2 ounces) white wine
- 1/2 cup (4 ounces) lemon juice
- 3 teaspoons (1/2 ounce) flour
- Pepper and salt

## Directions:

1. Pull out a medium sized skillet or pan and set the heat to medium.

2. While the pan heats up, dice your onion. Once the pan reaches the desired heat (do the water flick test to check), place the lard into it and let it melt a bit before adding the onions.

3. Cook the onions and lard until soft and they begin to turn a nice light brown color (you want to sweat the onions to bring out their sweetness).

4. Once the onions reach the perfect texture and color, toss them into your pressure cooker. Add the chicken breasts, minced garlic cloves, chicken broth, parsley, paprika, white wine, and lemon juice.

5. Place the lid on your pressure cooker and secure it tightly. Let the mixture cook for 10 minutes or until the chicken is cooked through (it may take up to 15 minutes).

6. If the sauce is too thin, add some of the flour to thicken it up until the desired thickness is reached.

7. Stir everything a few times to makes sure the ingredients are well combined. Serve hot or store in the refrigerator for reheating later.

## Extra tips for this recipe:

- Feel free to adjust the sauce after everything's been cooked. Simply ladle some from your pressure cooker, toss it into a medium skillet or saucepan and add flour to thicken. This works well if you want to drizzle a thick sauce over the top of your chicken.
- White wine works well with this recipe, but be sure to find something spicy to go with the spices in the chicken.
- The garlic makes the chicken versatile with a lot of Italian foods. Try serving the chicken on the side of a plate of spaghetti or other pasta.

# The Miraculous Chrysanthemum Flower

What few people care to consider when thinking about their diet and overall health is the benefits of tea and other herbal practices. Sure, they may seem a bit cliche and mystical, but many herbal teas and natural plants and flowers have amazing benefits to offer whoever ingests them. Among these plants and flowers is the miraculous Chrysanthemum flower.

Research focusing on the benefits and applications of herbal teas and flowers has been done, and the results are unbelievable by most people's' standards. While many flowers and herbs offer vary antioxidant benefits, the chrysanthemum has offered one peculiar additional benefit: Cholesterol reduction in those who ingest it on a normal basis.

Research shows that ingesting the chrysanthemum flower or a tea created from the flower has the ability to drastically reduce cholesterol levels even with a diet high in fat and cholesterol.

While not much is known about ingesting the flower and the full benefits that accompany it, one thing is certain above all out: There have been no apparent downsides to ingesting the flower. The worst thing that can come of drinking tea made from chrysanthemum is just that, the physical drinking of the tea itself (some people may find the tea too bitter).

As people spend more and more time and energy researching the benefits of teas, especially the benefits associated with the chrysanthemum flower, more and more positive effects come to life: Brain cells purification, hormones adjustment, and digestion are all improved noticeably when teas (especially the chrysanthemum) are ingested.

People have used tea in their everyday diets for thousands of years because of the benefits it provides. The chrysanthemum flower is one example and has come to light in recent years as one of the most potent and beneficial teas one can make.

# Conclusion

Thank you again for downloading this book!

I hope this book was able to help you to find a better understanding of both the Ketogenic and Paleo diets as well as introduce you to some fun and unique (as well as incredibly delicious) recipes that fit into either diet's guidelines.

The next step is to simply practice, practice, practice, and learn. You know the basics of the diets and some foods to cook that illustrate just how tasty the Keto and Paleo diets can be. Now it's time to go out and experiment with recipes, or search through your local grocery store for new and exciting low carb ingredients to use in your own home-made recipes.

Finally, if you enjoyed this book, then I'd like to ask you for a favor, would you be kind enough to leave a review for this book on Amazon? It'd be greatly appreciated!

Click here to leave a review for this book on Amazon!

Thank you and good luck!

# Francesca Bonheur

# *Ketogenic*

# COOKBOOK

RESET YOUR METABOLISM WITH THESE EASY, HEALTHY *and* DELICIOUS KETOGENIC, PALEO *and* PRESSURE COOKER...

**BEEF RECIPES**

© Copyright 2016 Francesca Bonheur - All rights reserved.

This document is geared towards providing exact and reliable information in regards to the topic and issue covered. The publication is sold with the idea that the publisher is not required to render accounting, officially permitted, or otherwise, qualified services. If advice is necessary, legal or professional, a practiced individual in the profession should be ordered.

- From a Declaration of Principles which was accepted and approved equally by a Committee of the American Bar Association and a Committee of Publishers and Associations.

In no way is it legal to reproduce, duplicate, or transmit any part of this document in either electronic means or in printed format. Recording of this publication is strictly prohibited and any storage of this document is not allowed unless with written permission from the publisher. All rights reserved.

The information provided herein is stated to be truthful and consistent, in that any liability, in terms of inattention or otherwise, by any usage or abuse of any policies, processes, or directions contained within is the solitary and utter responsibility of the recipient reader. Under no circumstances will any legal responsibility or blame be held against the publisher for any reparation, damages, or monetary loss due to the information herein, either directly or indirectly.

Respective authors own all copyrights not held by the publisher.

The information herein is offered for informational purposes solely, and is universal as so. The presentation of the information is without contract or any type of guarantee assurance.

The trademarks that are used are without any consent, and the publication of the trademark is without permission or backing by the trademark owner. All trademarks and brands within this book are for clarifying purposes only and are the owned by the owners themselves, not affiliated with this document.

# Table of Contents

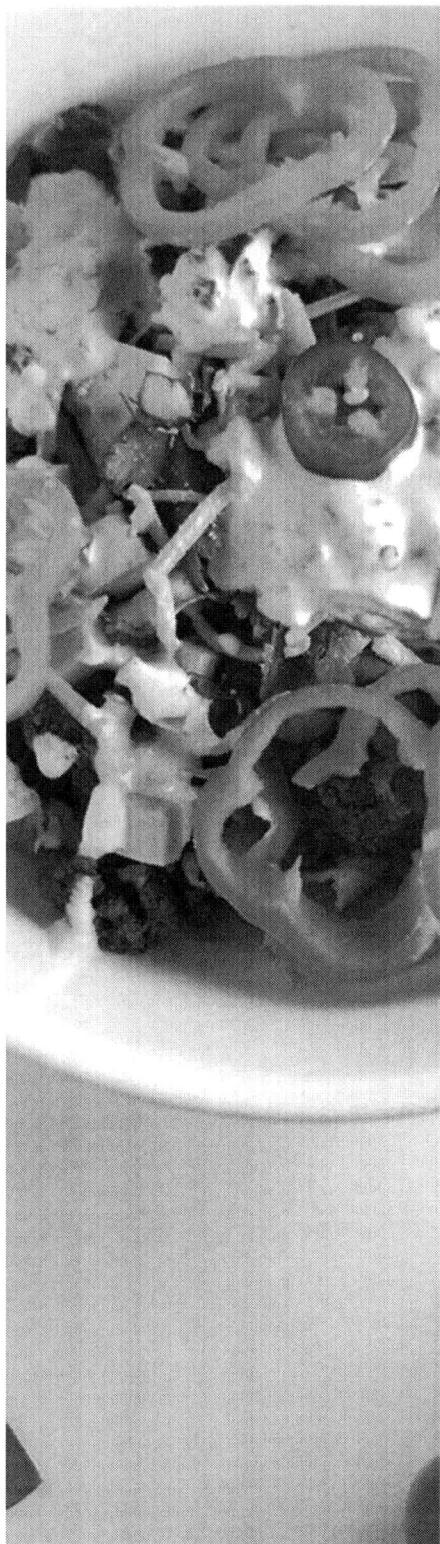

# Introduction

*I* want to thank you and congratulate you for downloading the book, *Ketogenic Cookbook.*

In this book, you are going to learn the various things that you are going to need to do in order to improve your diet and make yourself healthier with a newset of recipes that you may not have considered before.

This particular cookbook is going to be about the different beef recipes that there for a Ketogenic diet.

Thanks again for downloading this book, I hope you enjoy it!

Note: the nutritional information in this book is based per serving. I am not in any way a medical professional or even a nutritional professional and the nutritional information is placed in this book to assist those that may have other dietary needs that have to be monitored due to the advice of a medical professional.

Before you begin a keto diet, please talk to your doctor about any health issues that you may have that may be affected adversely by this diet.

Also be careful with this diet because it can end up causing some health issues if use improperly.

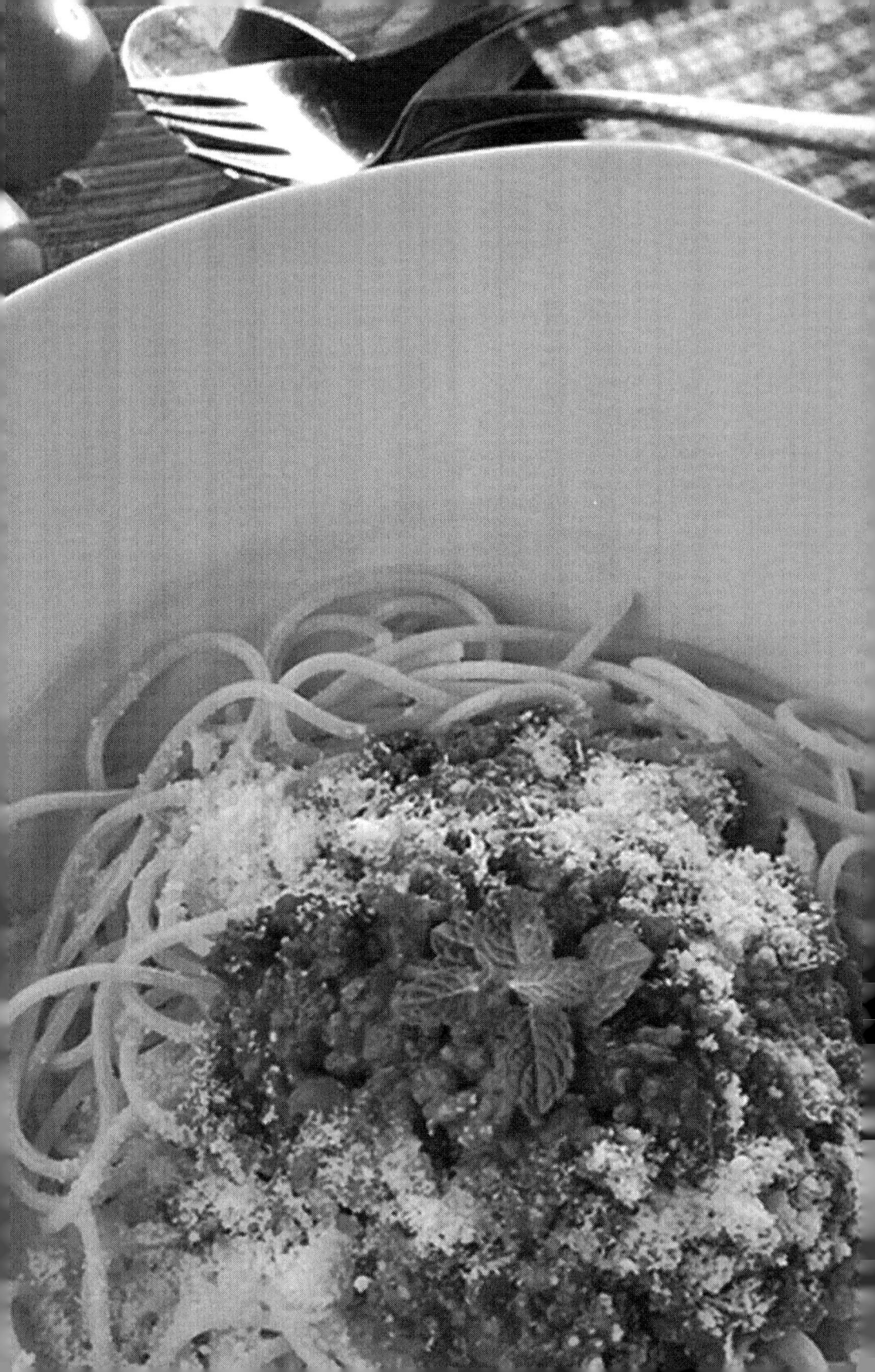

# CHAPTER
# 1

# The Ketogenic Diet

*W*hen you are using the keto diet, you are going to be following a diet that is high in fat, low in carbs, and gives you just enough protein. This is a diet that is highly effective when it comes to treating epilepsy in children.

With this diet, your body is going to be forced to burn the fat that is in your system at a faster rate than the carbohydrates are burned in your system. If you were not following this diet, your body would be taking the carbohydrates that are found in your food and turning it into glucose to be deposited around the body. But, if you do not have as many carbohydrates in your system, the body is forced to take the fat that is found in fatty foods and turn that into what the body needs.

In this diet, your body is going to reach a state called ketosis and the ketosis is going to assist in making your feel more energetic and healthier.

Some of the benefits of the Keto diet are:

1. Your body will be able to use the fat that is in your body to fuel your body so that you can keep going through the day which is not something that is going to happen if you are on a high carbohydrate diet. The more carbohydrates that your intake, the more energy you are going to feel, however when you have put your body into ketosis, then you are going to be forcing your body to become more efficient in fueling itself by using fats as energy.

2. With eating proteins less frequently, you are going to be making sure that you are taking in the proper qualities of protein that your body needs instead of overdoing it or underdoing it as so many people tend to do. At the point in time that you have forced your body into ketosis, you

are going to be wanting less food that is going to be turned into glucose in your system.

3. Now that your body does not have all of the insulin coursing through it, you are going to allow for your hormones to stabilize themselves when they are released into your body. Some of the hormones that are affected are the growth hormones.

4. While this is not as big of a benefit, it is still a benefit. The ketones that are going to be in your body now that you are in ketosis, you will find that you are no longer as hungry which is going to cause you to not eat as much!

Just like with any diet, there are going to be things that you can and cannot eat because they are going to do the opposite of what the diet is supposed to do. When you begin to diet, it can be frustrating trying to find things that are going to work for you that you enjoy. However, with the keto diet, you are not going to have that problem.

## Eat what you want

You can eat whatever you want on the keto diet for the most part. There are some things that you may not want to eat, however, there are not going to be many things.

## Wild animal and grass fed animals

- Meat that has been grass fed is going to be better for anyone anyways. Animals that are fed grass are going to be those that you find on a farm such as a goat, lamb, beef son on and so forth.
- Any fish that has been caught in the wild or any seafood but you are going to want to try and avoid any farmed fish.
- Pork and poultry that is pastured
- Gelatin
- Butter
- Ghee
- Pastured eggs

## Avoid

- Meat that is covered in breadcrumbs
- Sugary or starchy sauce meat

- Sausage
- Hot dogs
- The organ meats of grass fed animals such as the liver, kidneys, and heart.

## Fats that are healthy for you

### Saturated

- Lard
- Tallow
- Chicken fats
- Goose fats
- Duck fats
- Ghee
- Coconut oil
- Butter
- Clarified butter

### Monounsaturated

- Olive oil
- Avocado oil
- Macadamia oil

### Polyunsaturated

- Omega threes that are often found in seafood or fatty fish

## Vegetables that do not have starch

### Greens

- Lettuce
- Bok choy
- Swiss chard
- Chives
- Chard
- Spinach
- Radicchio
- Endive

## Cruciferous vegetables

- Kale (the dark leaf one is the best for you)
- Radishes
- Kohlrabi

## Other

- Cucumber
- Asparagus
- Celery stalks
- Summer squash
- Spaghetti squash
- Bamboo shoots
- Zucchini

## Fruit

- Avocado

## Condiments and beverages

- Water (of course because it is one of the healthiest things that you can drink!)
- Tea (black tea and herbal tea are the best)
- Coffee (do not put creamer in it, though. If you cannot drink it black, then put cream or coconut milk in it for sweetness)
- Pork rinds are best for when you need to do breading
- Any spices or herbs
- Lime juice and zest
- Lemon juice and zest
- Mustard
- Pesto
- Mayonnaise
- Pickles
- Bone broth (you are going to want to make your own so that you can control what goes in it.)
- Foods that are fermented (kimichi, sauerkraut (make your own) and kombucha)

- Whey proteins
- Egg whites

## Eat sparingly

Vegetables, fruits, mushrooms

- Red cabbage
- White cabbage
- Green cabbage
- Broccoli
- Cauliflower
- Fennel
- Rutabaga
- Brussels sprouts
- Parsley root
- Leek
- Mushroom
- Onion
- Garlic
- Spring onion
- Winter squash
- Eggplant
- Peppers
- Tomatoes
- Bean sprouts
- Okra
- Kombu
- Nori
- Coconut
- Rhubarb
- Olives
- Sugar snap peas
- French artichokes
- Wax beans
- Water chestnuts
- Blackberries

- Strawberries
- Blueberries
- Cranberries
- Raspberries
- Mulberries

Grain fed animals and dairy

- Ghee
- Eggs
- Poultry
- Beef
- Try and not eat pork that is farmed because it is too high in omega 6s.
- Bacon (it has a lot of starch and preservatives)
- Full fat yogurt
- Sour cream
- Cheese
- Cottage cheese
- Try and avoid things that are low fat!

Nuts and seeds

- Brazil nuts (however do not eat a lot of them because of the high levels of selenium they contain)
- Hemp seeds
- Sunflower seeds
- Macadamia nuts
- Walnuts
- Almonds
- Pine nuts
- Flaxseed
- Sesame seeds
- Pumpkin seeds

Soy products

Try and stick with non-GMO soy products if you have to eat them. Fermented soy products are good too.

- Soy sauce
- Natto

- Tempeh
- Coconut aminos that are paleo friendly
- Green soy beans
- Black soybeans

## Condiments

- Erythritol
- Swerve
- Stevia
- Arrowroot powder
- Xanthan gum
- Extra dark chocolate
- Carob powder
- Coco powder
- Ketchup
- Pureed tomatoes
- Passata tomatoes

Do not chew gum that is sugar free or suck on mints that are sugar free because where they do not have sugar, they have carbs.

## Vegetables and fruits

- Carrots
- Sweet potato
- Beetroot
- Parsnip
- Celery root
- Honeydew melon
- Galia melon
- Watermelon
- Cantaloupe
- Dragon fruit
- Apricot
- Peaches
- Cherries
- Pears
- Figs

- Plumbs
- Oranges
- Kiwi berries
- Kiwifruit
- Apples
- Nectarines
- Grapefruit

## Alcohol

- Unsweet spirits
- Dry white wine
- Dry red wine

## Avoid

These are the foods that you are going to want to avoid because they are meats that are factory farmed, food that is processed, and rich in carbohydrates.

## Grains

- Wholemeal
- Wheat
- Corn
- Rye
- Oats
- Millet
- Barley
- Bulgur
- Rice
- Sorghum
- Amaranth
- Rice
- Buckwheat
- Sprouted grains
- White potatoes
- Quinoa
- Pasta
- Pizza

- Cookies
- Bread
- Crackers
- Table sugar
- Ice cream
- Sweet pudding
- Agave syrup
- Soft drinks
- HFCS

## Factory farmed fish and pork

- Fish that is high in mercury
- Fish inflamed with omega 6
- Fish with PCBs

## Processed foods

- Food with carrageenan
- MSG
- BPAs
- Sulphites
- Artificial sweeteners
- Oils or fats that are refined
- Low carb products
- Zero carb products
- Low fat products
- Milk
- Sweet drinks
- Alcohol
- Tropical fruits
- Tropical fruit juices
- Tropical dried fruits
- Soy products (this is not just for the diet, but your health in general.)
- Wheat gluten
- Carrageenan

If you are unsure if you are allowed to eat it, you can either ask your doctor or do not eat it. Even if you think that it is okay to put into your diet, you may be harming yourself in the long run.

# Beef Breakfast Recipes

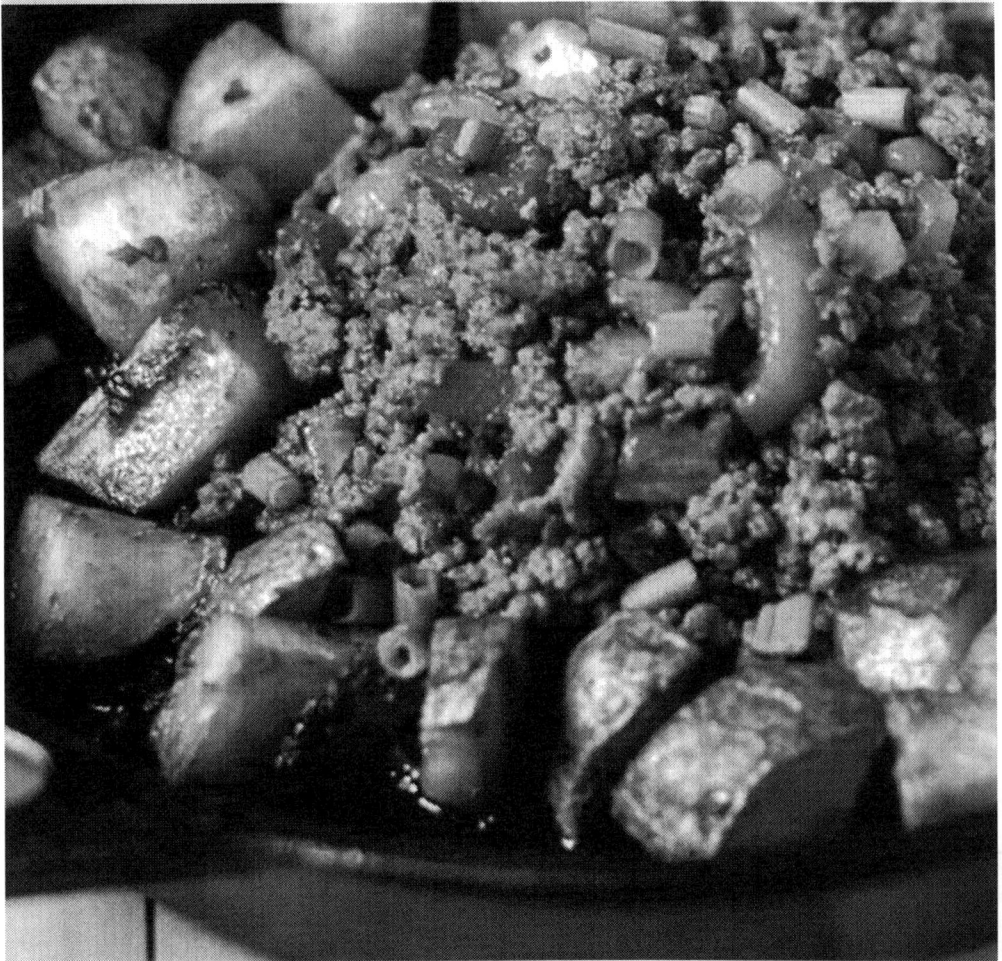

# Mug muffin with beef, mushrooms, and cheese

Prep time for this recipe is ten minutes while cook time is five minutes. You will end up with two servings.

## Ingredients:

- Salt (to taste)
- Flour (almond, 0.9 ounce)
- Water (2 tablespoons)
- Flaxmeal (1.3 ounces)
- Coconut milk or cream (2 tablespoons)
- Baking soda (0.25 teaspoon)
- Egg (1)
- Parsley (chopped)
- Basil (chopped)
- Ground beef (32 grams)
- Cheddar cheese (.5 cup)
- Mushrooms (.9 ounce)

## Directions:

1. Cook the beef until there is no pink.

2. Get rid of the liquid except for one tablespoon.

3. Cut the mushrooms up and cook them for about five minutes or until they are browned.

4. Take all of your dry ingredients and mix them into a bowl.

5. With a fork, mix in the cream, water, and egg until it is mixed well.

6. Combine the beef and mushrooms to the mixture.

7. Divide up into two mugs and add in any extras you may want.

8. Microwave for ninety seconds.

9. Let sit for five minutes.

10. Enjoy!

   Note: if you are wanting to cook it in the oven, cook it for fifteen minutes at 175 C (350 F)

## Nutritional Facts:

➟ 399 Milligrams Potassium
➟ 124 Milligrams Magnesium
➟ 434 Kilocalories
➟ 37.2 Grams Fat
➟ 18.7 Grams Protein
➟ 6.5 Grams Fiber
➟ 8.9 Grams Carbs

# Pizza beef frittata

Making this recipe from start to finish is going to take about twenty-five minutes. It will make up to four servings.

## Ingredients:

### Base

- Bell pepper (red, 1)
- Eggs (6)
- Onion(white, diced, 1)
- Marinara sauce (2.8 ounces)
- Ground beef (1 cup)
- Oregano (dried, .5 teaspoon)
- Ghee (1 tablespoon)
- Parmesan cheese (grated, 1.1 ounces)
- Mozzarella cheese (grated, 1.3 ounces)

### Topping

- Basil (fresh)
- Parmesan cheese (grated, 0.8 ounce)
- Pepperoni slices (28 grams)
- Mozzarella cheese (grated, 1 ounce)

## Directions:

1. Beat eggs in a bowl.
2. Mix in oregano, parmesan, marinara sauce, and mozzarella.
3. Use ghee to grease the pan and then cook your ground beef until it is no longer pink.
4. Throw the onion and bell pepper and cook until it is soft.
5. Dump the eggs into the pan and cook for around ten minutes.
6. Top off with cheese and slices of pepperoni.
7. Put in a broiler for about seven minutes.
8. Allow to cool before topping with basil and enjoying.

## Nutritional Facts:

- 4.9 Grams Carbs
- 296 Milligrams Potassium
- 1 Gram Fiber
- 31 Milligrams Magnesium
- 25.4 Grams Protein
- 426 Kilocalories
- 33.4 Grams Fat

# Beef and pumpkin breakfast casserole

Prep time for the beef and pumpkin casserole is twenty minutes while the total time is fifty minutes. It yields six servings.

## Ingredients:

- Salt and pepper (to taste)
- Ground beef (17.6 ounces)
- Ghee (1.6 ounces)
- Onion (white, 1)
- Heavy whipping cream (.5 cup)
- Garlic (3 cloves)
- Eggs (6)
- Pumpkin (diced, 8.2 ounces)
- Cheddar cheese (shredded, 8 ounces)
- Mustard or Dijon mustard (1 tablespoon)

## Directions:

1. Heat up the oven to 175 C (350 F).

2. Cook the beef in a pan that has been greased with ghee. Make sure to break any large pieces apart.

3. Cook until completely browned.

4. Place meat in a bowl and set aside.

5. Put the onion and the garlic in the pan and cook until lightly browned. This will be about ten minutes of your time.

6. Cut up the pumpkin and put in the pan and cook until it has become fork tender.

7. Once done, put in the bowl with the ground beef and add in mustard of your choosing.

8. Mix in cheese until well combined.

9. Crack and mix eggs with cream and season to taste with salt and pepper.

10. Place in a bowl.

11. Coat in egg mixture so every inch of the beef and pumpkin is covered.

12. Use what cheese you have left over to cover the top of the egg mix.

13. Cook for twenty-five minutes.

14. Serve with sriracha sauce.

## ❤ Nutritional Facts:

➡ 501 Milligrams Potassium
➡ 7.1 Grams Carbs
➡ 39 Milligrams Magnesium
➡ 1 Gram Fiber
➡ 577 Kilocalories
➡ 30.7 Grams Protein
➡ 47.3 Grams Fat

# Beef and egg stuffed pattypan squash

The total time you will spend making this recipe is forty-five minutes, twenty of which are going to be spent doing prep work. It is going to result in four servings.

## Ingredients:

- Salt and pepper (to taste)
- Pattypan squash (4)
- Eggs (4)
- Garlic (cloves, 2)
- Parmesan cheese (grated, 3 ounces)
- Onion (white, 1)
- Ground beef (1 cup)
- Ghee (1.9 ounces)

## Directions:

1. Turn the oven on to 175 C (350 F).

2. Cut the top off the squash and remove the guts.

3. Keep the guts in a bowl for later.

4. Cover the top of the squash with ghee that has been melted.

5. Put on a baking sheet and cook for twenty minutes. They should be fork tender when they come out.

6. Put the onion and garlic in a pan with the ghee that is left over and cook until they are brown. This is going to be about five minutes.

7. Cook the ground beef until it is brown. Be sure to stir the mixture so that it does not burn.

8. Take all the seeds from the guts that you took out of the squash. The soft seeds are okay to keep if you want so that you can roast them later on.

9.  After your beef is browned. Mix the squash guts in and cook for about five minutes.

10. If the parmesan is not already grated, go ahead and grate it.

11. Place the cheese in the pan and season to taste. Mix everything together until it is combined thoroughly.

12. Place the mixture into the squash and crack an egg on the inside of the squash to cover the beef mixture.

13. Cook for about twenty minutes or until the egg is done but the yolk is runny still.

14. Serve with crisp greens.

## ♥ Nutritional Facts:

➠ 546 Milligrams Potassium
➠ 19.9 Grams Protein
➠ 62 Milligrams Magnesium
➠ 31.4 Grams Fat
➠ 400 Kilocalories
➠ 10.7 Grams Carbs
➠ 2.7 Grams Fiber

# Mexican Breakfast Meatzza

This recipe takes 25 minutes to cook, 5 minutes to rest. You are going to get 8 servings out of it.

## Ingredients:

- Red onion (0.5 c diced)
- Ground beef (16 oz)
- Avocado large (1, diced)
- Mexican chorizo (16 oz)
- Tomato large (1, diced)
- Enchilada sauce (0.5 cup)
- Clarified butter or ghee (45 grams)
- White eggs large (8)
- Salt and pepper as desired

## Directions:

1. Heat oven to 176.6 degrees Celsius (350 F).

2. Combine chorizo and beef in a bowl.

3. Place on a cookie sheet or any other sheet that is shallow so there is uniformed thickness.

4. Place enchilada sauce across the meat.

5. Cook for 25 minutes. Be sure to turn the pan at the halfway mark. Meat needs to be fully cooked.

6. Remove any liquids that pooled in the pan.

7. Cool for 5 minutes.

8. Scramble eggs and ghee in a skillet until desired consistency is met.

9. Place over the pizza.

10. Equally distribute the seasoning, tomato, avocado and onion.

11. Enjoy!

## ❤ Nutritional Facts:

➡ 503 calories
➡ 0.6939 Grams Potassium (693.9 Grams)
➡ 0.04 Kilograms Fat (40 Grams)
➡ 0.0259 Kilograms Protein (25.9 Grams)
➡ 0.6868 Grams Sodium (686.8 Milligram)
➡ 0.0033 Kilogram Sugar (3.3 Grams)
➡ 0.2679 Gram Cholesterol (267.9 Milligram)
➡ 0.0098 Kilogram Carbohydrates (9.8 Grams)
➡ 0.0028 Kilogram Fiber (2.8 Grams)

# Grain Free Breakfast Taco Pie Filling

The prep time for this recipe is 30 minutes, cook time is 45 minutes which totals out to an hour and fifteen minutes. You are going to end up with one pie that has eight slices in it.

## Ingredients:

➡ Mango salsa (optional)
➡ Ground beef (grass fed, 340.194 grams or ¾ pound)
➡ Baking soda (0.3 tablespoons, 1 teaspoon)
➡ Taco seasoning (9 teaspoons, 3 tablespoons)
➡ Coconut oil (0.3 tablespoon, 1 teaspoon)
➡ Onion (white 0.5)
➡ Cilantro (to taste)
➡ Bell pepper (red, 0.5)
➡ Eggs (grass fed, 8)
➡ Sea salt (0.3 tablespoon, 1 teaspoon)

## Directions:

1. Cook the meat in the oil.
2. Once browned, add in seasonings to taste.
3. Remove juice.
4. Using the same pan, sauté onion and bell pepper together with juice you drained off the meat.
5. Mix eggs, baking soda, sea salt, and cilantro together.
6. Add more cilantro to onion and bell pepper.
7. Place in meat mix in pie crust.
8. Add in onion and bell pepper.
9. Top off with eggs.
10. Cook for 45 minutes at 176.6 C or 350 F.
11. Serve with salsa if so desired but enjoy!

# Dijon Beef Breakfast Skillet

This recipe is going to take 8 minutes to cook and will make 4 servings.

## Ingredients:

- Dijon mustard (6 teaspoons, 2 tablespoons)
- Ground beef (16 ounces, 1 pound)
- Basil (0.3 tablespoon, 0.5 teaspoon)
- Mushrooms (236.58 grams, 8 ounces, chopped coarsely)
- Salt (0.3 tablespoon, 0.5 teaspoon)
- Pepper (0.3 tablespoon, 0.5 teaspoon)
- Garlic powder (0.5 teaspoon)
- Zucchini (2, sliced into half-moons)

## Directions:

1. The oil needs to be cooked in a skillet.

2. Brown mushrooms for about four minutes.

3. Add in zucchini and season to taste cook until it is soft. (about four minutes).

4. Put vegetables on side of pan.

5. Add in meat and spices, break down meat into pieces.

6. Mix together with vegetables once fully cooked.

7. Add mustard and heat all the way through.

8. Season to taste.

## Nutritional Facts:

- 17 Carbs

# Deep dish beef breakfast casserole

For this recipe, you will cook it for 44 minutes and allow it to rest for about 10 minutes.

## Ingredients:

- Avocado oil (3 tablespoons)
- Ground beef (16 ounces, 1 pound)
- Eggs (10)
- Spinach (0.03 cup)
- Onion (1 medium diced)

## Directions:

1. Heat oil in skillet.

2. Brown beef for about four minutes.

3. Add in onion, proceed to sauté until translucent.

4. Turn oven on to 176.6C (350 F).

5. Drop spinach into mix until gone.

6. Cover dish with oil.

7. Place mixture into dish.

8. Pour eggs over the top (eggs should be beaten).

9. Mix together.

10. Cook for 30 minutes.

11. Cover the last 7 minutes so there is no burning.

12. Allow to cool for 10 minutes.

# Beef Breakfast Sausage

The cook time will be five minutes and it will yield as many as you want.

## Ingredients:

- Coconut oil (0.125 cup, 29.57 grams)
- Ground beef (grass fed, 48 ounces, 3 pounds)
- Onion powder (3 teaspoon, 1 tablespoon)
- Sage (dried, 59.147 grams, 0.25 cup)
- Sea salt (3 teaspoon, 1 tablespoon)

## Directions:

1. Combine all ingredients until evenly mixed.

2. Create burgers with your hands.

3. Melt choice of fat in skillet.

4. Fry for five minutes before flipping and frying or another five minutes.

   Note: Create small burgers because it will be saltier than regular beef.

# Beef Lunch Recipes

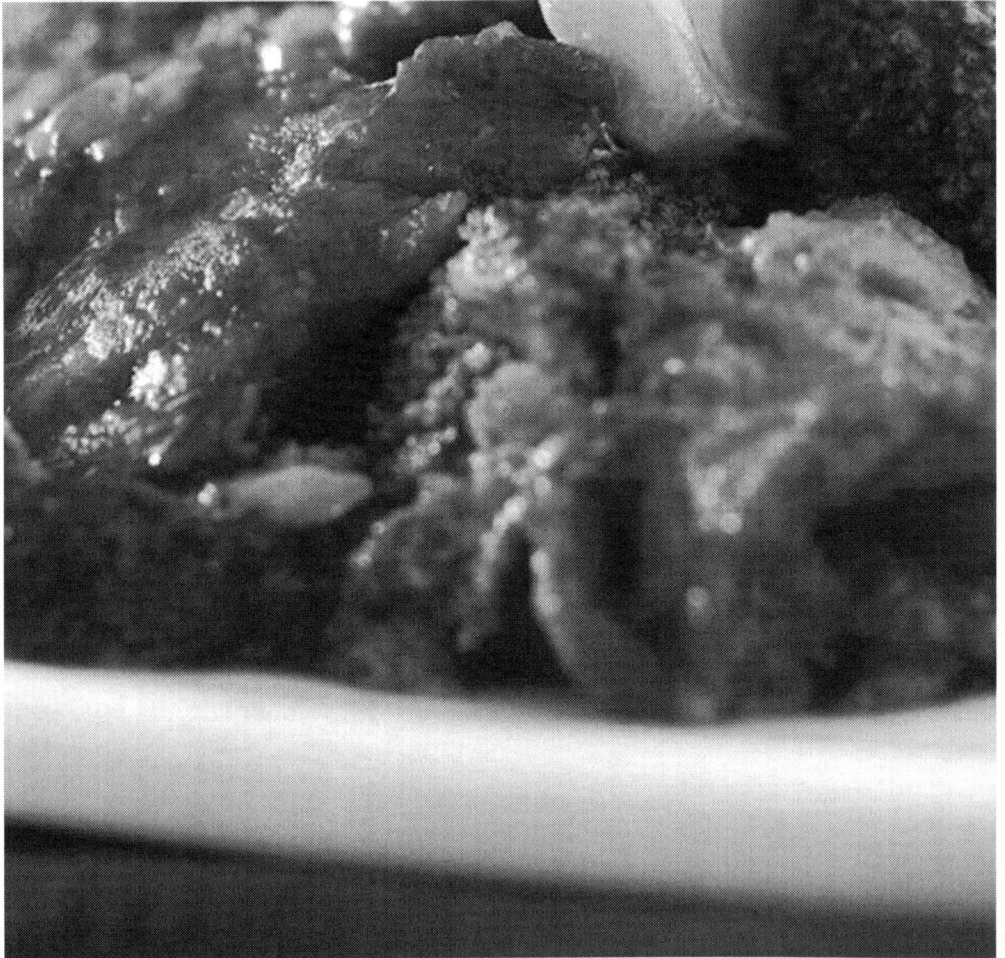

# Spaghetti squash Lasagna

The prep time for this recipe is 10 minutes, it takes 80 minutes to cook which is going to result in you spending an hour and thirty minutes on it. It yields around 12 servings

## Ingredients:

- Ground beef (48 ounces, 3 pounds)
- Mozzarella cheese (30 slices)
- Spaghetti squash (2 large)
- Marinara sauce (1133.98 grams, 40 ounces)
- Ricotta cheese (whole milk, 907.18 grams, 32 ounces)

## Directions:

1. Turn on the oven to 190.5 C (375 F).
2. Cut the squash in half and place face down in a pan of water.
3. Cook for 45 minutes until the skin can be peeled off.
4. Brown the meat in a skillet.
5. Place meat in saucepan and mix with marinara.
6. Once the squash is done, cut out squash guts.
7. Put lasagna in a pan that is greased (squash, meat, mozzarella, ricotta).
8. Do this until there is nothing left.
9. Cook for another 35 minutes or until bubbles.

## Nutritional Facts:

- 43 grams of Protein (0.0430 Kilograms)
- 711 Calories
- 2 Grams of Fiber (0.002 Kilograms)
- 59 Grams of Fat (0.0590 Kilograms)
- 15 Carbohydrates

# Spaghetti squash with meatballs

While preparing this recipe, you are going to spend 25 minutes on prep and an hour on cooking. It yields 10 servings.

## Ingredients:

### Meatballs

➡ Salt and pepper
➡ Ground beef (16 ounces)
➡ Egg (1)
➡ Onion (0.3)
➡ Cheddar cheese (shredded, 2 ounces)
➡ Pepper (green, 0.3)
➡ Garlic (minced, 1 tablespoon)
➡ Coconut flour (1 tablespoon)

### Spaghetti

➡ Marinara sauce (24 ounces)
➡ Spaghetti squash (1)
➡ Parmesan cheese (10 teaspoons)

## Directions:

1. Cut squash in half and gut.

2. Put in container with water.

3. Cook for 45 minutes at 190.5 C (375 F).

4. Cut pepper and onion.

5. Mix with beef, coconut flour, cheddar cheese, egg, and salt and pepper to taste.

6. Cut into around 10 meatballs.

7. Cook at 190.5 C for 25 minutes.

8. Place squash into a container.

9. Add meatballs to the squash.

10. Mix in tomato sauce.

11. Top with cheese.

## ❤ Nutritional Facts:

- 45 grams Protein
- 306 Calories
- 3 Grams Fiber
- 21 Grams Fat
- 13 Grams Carbohydrates

# Chili soup

This recipe calls for five minutes of prep and six hours of cooking. It yields around eight servings.

## Ingredients:

- Tomato paste (3 tablespoons)
- Butter (unsalted, 2 tablespoons)
- Coconut milk (unsweet, 0.25 cup)
- Onion (1)
- Beef stock (8 ounces)
- Pepper (1)
- Lemon juice (3 tablespoons)
- Ground pepper (16 ounces)
- Coconut flour (1 tablespoon)
- Bacon (8 slices, optional)
- Garlic (minced, 1 tablespoon)
- Thyme (1 tablespoon)
- Pepper (1 teaspoon)
- Salt (1 teaspoon)

## Directions:

1. Put butter in the center of the crockpot to melt.
2. Place onions and peppers in the bottom of the crockpot.
3. Place in ground beef.
4. Place bacon strips if you are using them.
5. Add in all seasonings.
6. Add in liquids.
7. Cover with tomato paste.
8. To cook, cover the pop and cook for about six hours.
9. Stir to mix everything together.
10. Top with cheese and enjoy.

## Nutritional Facts:

- 41 Grams of Protein
- 21 Grams of Fat
- 2 Grams of Fiber
- 396 Calories
- 7 Carbohydrates

# Keto taco salad

Prep time here is ten minutes, cook time is fifteen minutes resulting in twenty-five minutes being spent on making this meal that is going to make up to six servings.

## Ingredients:

- Cayenne pepper (to taste)
- Ground beef (2 pounds)
- Romaine leaf (6)
- Cheddar cheese (shredded, 1.125 cups)
- Salsa (12 tablespoons)
- Taco seasoning ( 6 tablespoons)
- Salsa (12 tablespoons)
- Sour cream (12 tablespoons)

## Directions:

1. Put meat in skillet and brown.

2. Add in taco seasonings and any other spices.

3. Cook until seasonings are mixed into the meat.

4. Cool and separate into containers.

5. Add in sour cream and salsa.

6. Add in romaine lettuce.

7. Enjoy!

## Nutritional Facts:

- 1 Gram of Fiber
- 38 Grams of Protein
- 647 Calories
- 5 Carbohydrates
- 51 Grams of Fat

# Mexican spinach casserole

To prep this recipe you will spend about fifteen minutes before allowing it to cook for forty-five minutes. There will be twelve servings when finished.

## Ingredients:

⇒ Spinach (drained, 2.5 cups)
⇒ Ground beef (32 ounces)
⇒ Jalapenos (optional)
⇒ Rotel (drained, 2 cans)
⇒ Taco seasoning (4 teaspoons)
⇒ Mozzarella cheese (shredded, 1 cup)
⇒ Cream cheese (2 cups)
⇒ Onion (medium, 1)
⇒ Sour cream (10 tablespoons)
⇒ Pepper (green, 1)

## Directions:

1. Cook onions and pepper after dicing them. They should be translucent.

2. Add in jalapenos if desired.

3. Place in a bowl.

4. Cook spinach until thawed if frozen, get rid of as much moisture from spinach as possible.

5. Place in prep bowl with vegetables.

6. Cook meat until brown.

7. Cook in taco seasoning.

8. Move to bowl.

9. Add in rotel after draining.

10. Add in sour cream, cream cheese, and mozzarella and mix thoroughly.

11. Place in a large pan (9 x 13).

12. Cook for 40 minutes at 176.6 C (350 F).

## ♥ Nutritional Facts:

⇒ 11 Carbohydrates
⇒ 403 Calories
⇒ 26 Grams Protein
⇒ 27 Grams Fat
⇒ 3 Grams Fiber

# Beef and broccoli

Enjoy your Chinese food? Well, why not make it at home! All it takes is ten minutes for prepping, an hour for margination, and then eight minutes to cook. Seems easy enough right? Plus, you are going to end up with four servings!

## Ingredients:

- Flank steak (cut into strips, 24 ounces)
- Baking soda (.5 teaspoon)
- Oil (vegetable, 2 tablespoons)
- Sugar (1 teaspoon)
- Water (1 tablespoon)
- Cornstarch (1 tablespoon)
- Soy sauce (low-sodium is best, 1 tablespoon)
- Broccoli (2 heads, crowns only)
- Soy sauce (low sodium, .5 cup)
- Oil (vegetable, 3 tablespoons)
- Brown sugar (2 tablespoons)
- Sherry (1 tablespoon)
- Garlic (minced, 4 cloves)
- Flour (2 tablespoons)

## Directions:

1. You need to marinate the meat first. In order to do this, you are going to combine the vegetable oil, water, soy sauce, cornstarch, sugar, baking soda, together in a bowl (first six ingredients).

2. Place meat into the marinade and shake to coat the meat.

3. Cover and place in the fridge for an hour.

4. Mix soy sauce, flour, garlic, brown sugar, and sherry in a bowl until it is completely smooth.

5.  In a wok or saute pan, heat up the vegetable oil.

6.  Saute the broccoli for three minutes.

7.  Remove and reduce heat.

8.  Place last of oil in the pan.

9.  Put in the meat and half the sauce it sat in and cook for 4 minutes stirring to avoid burning.

10. Make sure there is no pink in the meat.

11. Mix in the sauce and broccoli.

12. Cook for one more minute.

13. Enjoy!

# Cheesy cauliflower shepherd's pie

Serves eight.

## Ingredients:

### Filling

- Rosemary (fresh, chopped, 2 tablespoons)
- Ground lamb (16 ounces)
- Arrowroot starch (1 tablespoon)
- Ground beef (16 ounces)
- Red wine (dry, .5 cup)
- Onion (chopped, .5 cup)
- Garlic (minced, 1 clove)
- Salt (1 teaspoon)
- Pepper (.5 teaspoon)

### Topping

- Cheddar cheese (grated, .5 cup)
- Cauliflower (24 ounces)
- Pepper (.25 teaspoon)
- Garlic (2 cloves)
- Salt (.5 teaspoon)
- Butter (2 tablespoons)

## Directions:

### Filling

1. Brown the meat for about twelve minutes.

2. Place in a bowl.

3. Get rid of all the liquid in the pan except for a tablespoon.

4. Reheat the pan and add in pepper, onion, and salt. Cook until onions are translucent.

5. Throw in garlic.

6. Mix in meat.

7. Stir starch into wine and add to the pan.

8. Cook until wine is almost gone and juice is thick.

9. Stir in rosemary.

10. Take off heat and put in a casserole dish.

*Topping*

1. Heat the oven to 204 C (400 F).

2. Place a basket for steaming into a stock pot with water.

3. Steam the garlic and cauliflower for around eight minutes.

4. Drain well and place in a food processor.

5. Throw in the salt, pepper, and butter and mix until smooth.

6. Put in the casserole dish.

7. Sprinkle with cheese.

8. Bake for twenty-five minutes or until cheese has melted.

9. Turn your broiler on and broil for around four minutes so that the cheese is browned.

### Nutritional Facts:

- 659 Milligrams Sodium
- 413 Kilocalories
- 30.05 Grams Protein
- 1.32 Grams Polyunsaturated Fatty Acids
- 2.32 Grams Dietary Fiber
- 24.74 Grams Fat
- 8.42 Grams Carbohydrates
- 115 Milligrams Cholesterol
- 222 Calories from Fat

# Beef Dinner Recipes

# Mongolian beef

You are going to get two servings out of this recipe.

## Ingredients:

- Corn starch (2 teaspoons)
- Flank steak (sliced, 16 ounces)
- Brown sugar (.5 cup)
- Garlic (minced, 5 cloves)
- Soy sauce (.5 cup)
- Jalapeno (diced and seeded, 1)
- Oil (canola, 1 tablespoon)
- Ginger (peeled, diced, 1)
- Scallions (sliced, 5)

## Directions:

1. Coat the beef in a bowl with cornstarch.

2. Combine soy sauce, cornstarch (2 teaspoons), and brown sugar in a pan after mixing well.

3. Simmer mixture before lowering heat and stirring to avoid burning.

4. Heat oil in skillet.

5. Throw in ginger and jalapeno. Cook till the ginger is brown.

6. Add meat and garlic spreading it out over the pan evenly.

7. Cook until meat has no pink.

8. Cover in a sauce that the meat sat in. Mix until everything is thoroughly covered in sauce.

9. Pull off heat and mix in scallions.

10. Serve with rice!

# Keto taco cups

Prep time is ten minutes while cook time is fifteen minutes. It serves five.

## Ingredients:

### Fat head nacho cups

- Chili powder (to taste)
- Mozzarella (shredded, 6 ounces )
- Coriander powder (1 teaspoon)
- Flour (almond, 3 ounces)
- Cumin powder (1 teaspoon)
- Cream cheese (2 tablespoons)
- Salt (to taste)
- Egg (1)

### Beef mix

- Tomato paste (1 tablespoon)
- Onion (sliced, 1)
- Chili powder (.5 teaspoon)
- Tomatoes (canned, sliced, 14 ounces)

### Sides (optional)

- Sour cream
- Salad
- Avocado
- Guacamole
- Mozzarella (shredded)
- Salsa

## Directions:

### Meat mix

1. Fry the onion until they become clear.
2. Add in broken up meat and cook until completely brown.

3. Mix in the spices, canned tomatoes, and tomato paste.

4. Cook for fifteen minutes without a cover.

*Taco cups*

1. Combine cheese, flour in bowl.

2. Throw in cream cheese and microwave for a minute.

3. Stir and cook for another thirty seconds.

4. Pull out, stir, add spices and egg to mix.

5. Place on a baking sheet between two pieces of parchment paper.

6. Create circles with the dough using a cookie cutter or glass.

7. Move each cup to a muffin tin.

8. Cook for fifteen minutes at 220 C (425 F).

9. Pull out of tin and bake for 2 more minutes on parchment paper.

10. Put it together.

11. Put on a plate and create your cup.

12. Enjoy with your favorite sides.

   Note: you can also use coconut flour.

## Nutritional Facts:

- 9.7 Grams Carbohydrates
- 511 Calories
- 38.4 Grams Protein
- 35.6 Grams Fat

# Keto kitchen sink casserole

For thirty-five minutes you will be prepping before cooking for forty minutes. In the end, you are going to have twelve servings.

## Ingredients:

- Paprika (optional, to taste)
- Ground beef (9 cups)
- Cream cheese (2 cups)
- Onion (small, 1)
- Cheddar cheese (shredded, 1 cup)
- Celery (4 stalks)
- Bacon (7 slices)
- Sausage (3 cups)
- Cauliflower (froze, 2 cups)
- Mushrooms (sliced, 2 cups)

## Directions:

1. At 204.4 C (400 F) cook the bacon for about twenty minutes.

2. Prep the rest of the meal during this time.

3. Make sure the ground beef is broken up.

4. Cook in a pan until no pink is found.

5. Brown sausage.

6. Place in a bowl without the grease.

7. Cut up the onion and celery.

8. Place in the grease and cook until translucent.

9. Unfreeze the cauliflower by cooking and then slice up.

10. Add to a large bowl.

11. Add meat to bowl after draining liquid.

12. Add bacon once done.

13. Mix in cream cheese.

14. Add cheese before mixing again.

15. Place in pan and sprinkle with paprika if you want.

16. Cook for thirty minutes at 176.6 C (350 F) be sure it is covered.

17. Uncover and cook for another 10 minutes.

♥ Nutritional Facts:

➡ 52 Grams Protein
➡ 5 Carbohydrates
➡ 598 Calories
➡ 40 Grams Fat
➡ 1 Gram Fiber

# Cheesy beef casserole

For fifteen minutes you will be prepping for this meal and then it is going to take about twenty-five minutes to cook. In the end, you are going to end up with eight servings.

## Ingredients:

- Green onions (4 stalks)
- Ground beef (16 ounces)
- Salsa (green, 2 cups)
- Sour cream (8 ounces)
- Taco seasoning (4 teaspoons)
- Monterey Jack cheese (1 cup)
- Green chilies (diced, .5 cup)

## Directions:

1. Cut up ground beef.
2. Cook until there is no pink left.
3. Drain liquid.
4. Add in taco seasoning.
5. Move into a pan that has been greased.
6. Mix salsa, chili, sour cream and put over beef.
7. Cook for around twenty-five minutes at 176.6 C (350 F).
8. Add cheese before cooking for another five minutes.
9. Cool and place green onions on top.

## Nutritional Facts:

- 7 Carbohydrates
- 351 Calories
- 34 Grams Protein
- 17 Grams Fat
- 1 Grams Fiber

# Cabbage fradiavolo with beef

This recipe will take you a grand total of twenty-five minutes to make. Ten minutes are going to be spent prepping while another fifteen is going to be spent on the food cooking. Once it is done, you are going to have about eight servings to share with your friends and family.

## Ingredients:

- Ground beef (3 cups)
- Cabbage (green, 1 head)
- Salt and pepper to taste
- Butter (1 stick, unsalted)
- Pasta sauce (3 cups)
- Water (.5 cup)

## Directions:

1. Take apart the cabbage and throw away the outer layers.

2. Slice into quarters and place in a food processor to shred. (If you do not want to do this, then by cabbage that has already been shredded).

3. Put the butter in a pot and melt it down before adding the water and cabbage in along with the pepper and salt.

4. Cook for around twelve minutes, make sure to stir as to avoid burning.

5. Brown the beef while the cabbage is cooking and drain away all liquids.

6. Place beef in the cabbage pot and mix together.

7. Add pasta sauce in and mix once more.

8. Top with cheese if you want.

## Nutritional Facts:

- 19 Grams Protein
- 28 Grams Fat
- 365 Calories
- 11 Grams Carbohydrates
- 5 Grams Fiber

# Mexican spinach casserole

For fifteen minutes you will be prepping the ingredients for this meal before allowing it to cook for forty-five minutes. It serves twelve.

## Ingredients:

- Spinach (drained, 2.5 cups)
- Ground beef (32 ounces)
- Jalapenos (optional)
- Rotel (drained, 2 cans)
- Taco seasoning (4 teaspoons)
- Mozzarella cheese (shredded, 1 cup)
- Cream cheese (2 cups)
- Onion (medium, 1)
- Sour cream (10 tablespoons)
- Pepper (green, 1)

## Directions:

1. Take the pepper and onion and dice them.

2. Cook in oil until they become translucent.

3. Add jalapeno if desired.

4. Place onions and pepper in bowl.

5. Add in spinach after it has been cooked or thawed. You do not want any moisture in it if you can accomplish that, but a little is not going to harm it.

6. Brown meat.

7. Add in taco seasoning to the meat.

8. Move meat to the bowl with the pepper and onion.

9. Remove liquid from the rotel and add to mixture.

10. Mix in cream cheese, sour cream, and mozzarella.

11. Put in a baking dish (9x13 works best).

12. Cook for 40 minutes at 176.6 C (350 F).

## ♥ Nutritional Facts:

➠ 11 Grams Carbohydrates
➠ 403 Calories
➠ 26 Grams Protein
➠ 3 Grams Fiber
➠ 27 Grams Fat

# Almond bun personal pizzas

Prep time is ten minutes, cook time is twenty-five and it will yield three servings.

## Ingredients:

- Cheddar cheese (0.0625 cup)
- Almond buns (2)
- Ground beef (1 cup)
- Pizza sauce (4 tablespoons)
- Parmesan cheese (0.0625 cup)
- Mozzarella cheese (0.125 cup)

## Directions:

1. Make the almond buns (recipe can be found online).
2. Once done, put so that the flat side is facing up. This is the top of your pizza.
3. Evenly place the pizza sauce over the bun.
4. Add on your toppings.
5. Add a layer of cheese.
6. Add more toppings if desired.
7. The cheese needs to be melted and this will take about five minutes and toppings are crisp.

## Nutritional Facts:

- 27 Grams Protein
- 653 Calories
- 4 Grams Fiber
- 56 Grams Fat
- 10 Grams Carbohydrates

# Bacon cheeseburger casserole

The total time for this recipe is forty-five minutes. Twenty of which are used for prep time and the remaining thirty-five are used for cooking. It makes twelve servings which is enough to share or have left overs!

## Ingredients:

- Cheddar cheese (grated, 1.5 cups)
- Ground beef (32 ounces)
- Pepper (grounded, .25 teaspoon)
- Garlic (2 cloves)
- Salt (.5 teaspoon)
- Onion powder (.5 teaspoon)
- Heavy cream (8 ounces)
- Bacon (cooked and chopped, (16 ounces)
- Tomato paste (.75 cups)
- Eggs (8)

## Directions:

1. Cook the meat with the garlic and onion until it is browned.
2. Remove grease and place on the bottom of a pan.
3. Mix in pieces of bacon.
4. Whisk eggs, heavy cream, pepper, salt, and tomato paste together.
5. Mix in cheese to the mixture.
6. Cover meat with mix.
7. Top off with cheese.
8. Cook for thirty five minutes at 176.6C (350 F).

   Note: you can always reduce egg and add in more meat as well as other stuff such as onions, pickles, or anything else that you are wanting to add into it.

## Nutritional Facts:

- 548 Calories
- 48.5 Grams of Protein
- 365.6 Grams Total Fat
- 4.4 Grams Carbohydrates
- 262 Milligrams Cholesterol
- 1255 Milligrams Sodium

# Cuban beef in a crock pot

Prep time: 15 minutes, cook time: 6 hours, serves: 4

## Ingredients:

- Lime (1)
- Beef (chunk roast, 32 ounces)
- Cilantro (chopped, .5 cup)
- Cauliflower rice (32 ounces)
- Garlic (1 tablespoon)
- Poblano pepper (chopped, 1)
- Oregano (1 tablespoon)
- Onion (white, 1, half sliced thin, half chopped)
- Cumin (2 tablespoons)
- Tomato paste (0.75 cup)
- Oil (olive, 2 tablespoons)
- Beef broth (8 ounces)
- Paprika (smoked, 1 tablespoon)

## Directions:

1. Put oil in pan and heat to simmer.

2. Cook beef 2 minutes each side.

3. Put everything from the pan in your crockpot.

4. Add in everything but rice, lime, cilantro, and chopped onion.

5. Stir and cook for six hours.

6. When done, it should fall apart by using a fork.

7. Shred and cook for another thirty minutes.

8. Serve with rice, lime, onion, and cilantro.

# Beef Snacks

# Beef and bacon rolls

The prep time for these rolls is ten minutes with a cook time of three minutes. It will make up to four servings.

## Ingredients:

⇒ Steak seasoning (to taste)
⇒ Beef (2 cups)
⇒ Bacon (4 slices)

## Directions:

1. Heat oil in deep fryer to a temperature of 187.7 C (370 F).

2. Cut the beef into cubes (about 1" x 1" x 2").

3. Cut bacon slices into four equal strips.

4. Season to taste.

5. Wrap bacon around the beef and place a tooth pick through it.

6. Cook for around three minutes in the fryer.

7. Enjoy!

## Nutritional Facts:

⇒ 29 Grams Protein
⇒ 10 Grams Fat
⇒ 73 Milligrams Cholesterol
⇒ 215 Calories
⇒ 0 Grams Fiber
⇒ 0 Grams Carbohydrates
⇒ 251 Milligrams Sodium
⇒ 0 Grams Trans Fat
⇒ 4 Grams Saturated Fat
⇒ 0 Grams Unsaturated Fat

# Cheesy beef balls

The prep time is ten minutes, the cook time is five, and it yields around twelve servings based on this recipe.

## Ingredients:

→ Cheddar (cubed, 12, optional)
→ Ground beef (1.5 cups)
→ Cheddar cheese (shredded, 0.75 cup)

## Directions:

1. Combine the beef and the cheese.

2. Roll into twelve balls of equal size.

3. If you are placing the cubed cheese in the middle, make sure that you do this before you roll them into balls.

4. You can freeze the balls if you are not going to eat them right away.

5. When you get ready to cook them, deep fry them at 190.5 C (375 F).

## Nutritional Facts:

→ 0 Grams of Fiber
→ 12 Grams of Fat
→ 173 Calories
→ 10 Grams Protein

# Spicy beef cauliflower

There is not really anything that you are going to need to prep for this dish so you are only going to have to wait twenty five minutes for it to cook before you can enjoy it. It is going to yield four servings.

## Ingredients:

⇒ Old Bay seasoning (to taste)
⇒ Cauliflower (frozen, 2 cups)
⇒ Ground beef (1 cup)

## Directions:

1. Cook the frozen cauliflower in the microwave as the instructions state.

2. Brown the meat until there is no pink left.

3. Remove the meat from the pan.

4. Leaving the grease in the pan, add the cauliflower and cover with seasoning.

5. Sauté for about five minutes.

6. Reapply seasonings.

7. Mix until the cauliflower is thoroughly cooked and broken up into small pieces.

8. Add the meat to the mixture.

9. Mix together and enjoy.

## Nutritional Facts:

⇒ 6 Grams of Protein
⇒ 100 Calories
⇒ 6 Grams of Fat
⇒ 3 Grams Fiber
⇒ 5 Grams Carbohydrates

# Beef brussels sprouts

The time you spend prepping is going to be ten minutes and it is going to take about forty minutes to cook. You will end up with four serving sizes if you follow this recipe.

## Ingredients:

- Pepper (to taste)
- Brussels sprouts (3 cups)
- Ground beef (2 cups)
- Fish sauce (2 ounces)
- Oil or bacon grease (2 ounces)

## Directions:

1. Take the steams out of the brussels sprouts and cut them into quarters.

2. Mix the sprouts into the oil or bacon grease and fish sauce.

3. Cook the ground beef until there is no pink left.

4. Add this into the mixture along with your seasoning.

5. Place in a pan that has been greased.

6. For forty minutes, cook at 232.2 C (450 F).

7. Be sure you are stirring them every ten minutes.

8. After this is done, boil them for a few minutes before enjoying.

## Nutritional Facts:

- 6 Grams Protein
- 143 Calories
- 3 Grams Fiber
- 10 Grams Fat
- 8 Carbohydrates

# Mini pepper nachos

Serves six

## Ingredients:

⟶ Tomato (chopped, .5 cup)
⟶ Chili powder (1 tablespoon)
⟶ Cheddar cheese (shredded (1.5 cups)
⟶ Cumin (ground, 1 teaspoon)
⟶ Mini peppers (seeded, halved, 16 ounces)
⟶ Garlic powder (1 teaspoon)
⟶ Ground beef (16 ounces)
⟶ Paprika (1 teaspoon)
⟶ Red pepper flakes (.25 teaspoon)
⟶ Salt (kosher, .5 teaspoon)
⟶ Oregano (.5 teaspoon)
⟶ Pepper (.5 teaspoon)

## Directions:

1. Mix seasonings together in a bowl.

2. On medium heat, brown the meat (about ten minutes) be sure all the clumps are broken up.

3. Mix in the spices and continue to saute until the seasoning has gone through all of the meat.

4. Heat the oven to 204 C (400 F).

5. Put aluminum foil in the bottom of a tray.

6. Place the peppers in a single line. They can touch. The closer they are, the more you can get on the pan.

7. Coat with beef mix.

8. Sprinkle with cheese.

9. Bake for around ten minutes or until your cheese has melted.

10. Pull out of the oven and top with the toppings of your choice.

11. Enjoy!

## ♥ Nutritional Facts:

➡ 2.39 Grams Dietary Fiber Total
➡ 96 Milligrams of Cholesterol
➡ 28.41 Grams Protein (per serving)
➡ 31 KiloCalories
➡ 6.58 Grams Carbohydrates
➡ 21.97 Grams Fat Total

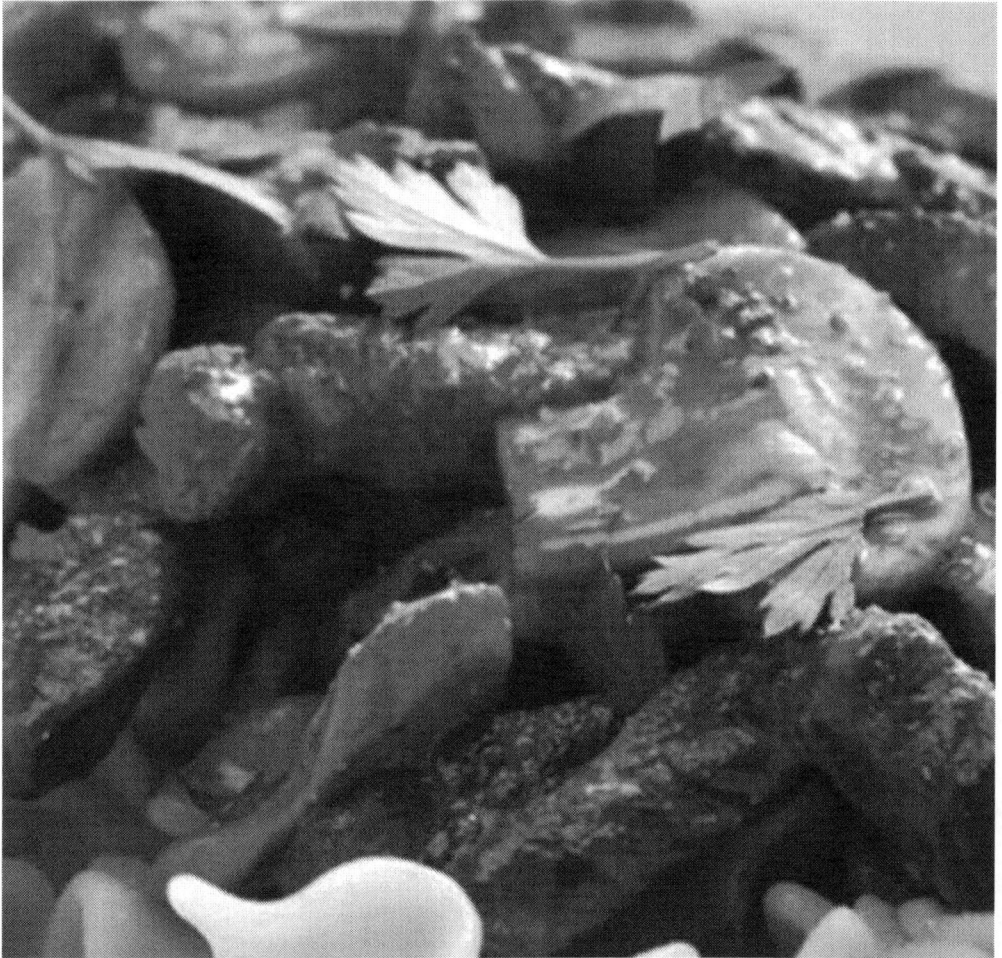

CHAPTER
**6**

# Beef Pressure Cooker Recipes

# Moroccan beef and cauliflower

Prep time is fifteen minutes and cook time is fifty five minutes. It yields up to four servings.

## Ingredients:

- Turmeric (0.25 teaspoon)
- Cauliflower (head, 1)
- Salt (.5 teaspoon)
- Beef (stew meat, 24 ounces)
- Pepper (.5 teaspoon)
- Olive oil (0.33 ounce)
- Ginger (.5 teaspoon)
- Onion (diced, .5)
- Cumin (0.16 ounce)
- Garlic (cloves, 2)
- Bouillion cube (beef, 1)
- Parsley (chopped, 0.25 cup)
- Tomato paste (0.16 ounce)

## Directions:

1. Take off the leaves that are on the head of cauliflower. Break the cauliflower into large pieces.
2. Rinse and put into a bowl.
3. Place olive oil in pressure cooker and heat it up.
4. Place stew meat in the oil and cook until there is no pink.
5. Add water to pot so that it covers the meat.
6. Place all ingredients except cauliflower into the pot.
7. Cover and cook for about fifteen minutes in the pressure cooker.
8. Coat cauliflower with sauce in pressure cooker.
9. Cover and let cook for another seven minutes or until the cauliflower is done.

## Nutritional Facts:

- 65.2 Grams of Protein
- 935.6 Calories
- 15.2 Grams Carbohydrates
- 841.8 Milligram Sodium
- 236.2 Milligram Cholesterol

# Beef stew with mushrooms

If you are wanting to make this recipe, you are going to spend ten minutes prepping and an hour allowing it to cook.

## Ingredients:

- Thyme (2 sprigs)
- Tomatoes (diced, 1.875 cups)
- Chicken stock (8 ounces)
- Red wine (.5 cup)
- Salt (kosher, 1 teaspoon)
- Mushrooms (sliced, 1 cup)
- Tomato paste (2 tablespoons)
- Garlic (minced, 3 cloves)
- Carrot (diced and peeled, 1)
- Celery (diced, 1 stalk)
- Onions (diced, 2)
- Salt kosher (2 tablespoons)
- Beef (2" cubes, 48 ounce)
- Vegetable oil (1 teaspoon)

## Directions:

1. Cook the meat in two different batches with the 2 teaspoons of salt.

2. Place the vegetable oil in the pressure cooker on medium high heat.

3. Add in half the meat and seat until there is no pink, do this for both batches of meat it will take about 3 minutes.

4. Once the meat is cooked, place it in a bowl.

5. Place the vegetables, tomato paste and garlic into pot.

6. Cover with last bit of salt.

7. Cook for eight minutes or until your onions are no longer crunchy.

8. Mix the red wine in allowing the pot to come to a simmer.

9. Stir making sure to get any meat that may be on the bottom of the pot so that it gets mixed into the mixture.

10. Add in beef and liquid that may have pooled in the bowl.

11. Add in the rest of the ingredients.

12. Cover and cook for around thirty minutes depending on your pressure cooker.

13. Once it is done, throw away the thyme sprig.

14. Season to taste.

15. Enjoy!

# Beef stroganoff

Prep time is ten minutes, cook time is thirty, and it makes six servings.

## Ingredients:

⇒ Traditional beef stroganoff calls for egg noodles, instead substitute it for your favorite vegetable such as spaghetti squash (1.5 cups)
⇒ Beef (cubed, 56 ounces)
⇒ Sour cream (1 cup)
⇒ Olive oil (2 tablespoons but you may need more)
⇒ Red wine (0.25 cup)
⇒ Flour (0.75 cup)
⇒ Beef stock (1.25 cups)
⇒ Salt (kosher, 1 teaspoon)
⇒ Garlic (minced, 3 cloves)
⇒ Pepper (.5 teaspoon)
⇒ Onion (sliced, 1)
⇒ Onion powder (.5 teaspoon)
⇒ Paprika (0.125 teaspoon)
⇒ Thyme (dried, .5 teaspoon)
⇒ Rosemary (dried, .5 teaspoon)

## Directions:

1. Mix together the seasonings in a zip lock bag.

2. Add in beef and shake until thoroughly coated.

3. Put in pressure cooker and allow to brown.

4. Add in oil.

5. You may need to do the meat in batches as to not overcrowd the pressure cooker and to ensure that all of the meat is being cooked properly.

6. When the beef has browned, remove it and put in the next batch until all the meat is cooked.

7. Place onions and more oil in allowing the onions to cook for about five minutes.

8. Next add in the garlic.

9. Replace the meat and any juices that may have collected on your plate.

10. Add beef stock and wine to the mixture.

11. Cover and cook for twenty minutes.

12. Place the sour cream in a bowl.

13. Move some of the juice from the pressure cook to the bowl with the sour cream and stir until mixed and the sour cream has become warm.

14. Now stir this into the meat mixture.

15. Season to taste.

16. Serve over your vegetable noodles that you made earlier.

# Meatloaf

Eight servings of meatloaf made in a pressure cook! It takes fifteen minutes to make and thirty to allow to cook before you are allowed to enjoy it!

## Ingredients:

- Beef stock (.5 cup)
- Ketchup or BBQ sauce (8 ounces)
- Onion (yellow, diced, 1)
- Oil (vegetable, 1 tablespoon)
- Pepper (.5 teaspoon)
- Salt (1 teaspoon)
- Thyme (dried, .5 teaspoon)
- Worcestershire sauce (2 teaspoons)
- Garlic (minced, 1 tablespoon)
- Egg (beaten 1)
- Parmesan cheese (grated, 0.25 cup)
- Onion (yellow, minced, 0.25 cup)
- Bread crumbs (Italian, .5 cup)
- Ground beef (16 ounces)

## Directions:

1. Mix seasonings, egg, onion that was minced, cheese, meat, and bread-crumbs into a bowl.

2. Create a loaf that is roughly the size of your pressure cooker.

3. Heat oil.

4. Saute onions in pressure cooker.

5. Add in ketchup (or BBQ sauce), beef stock.

6. Place meatloaf in.

7. Cook for 15 minutes.

# Glossary

When you are learning about the keto diet, there are going to be terms that you are going to hear that you may not know what they mean. This part of the book is going to be the part that is going to help you to understand all of those hard to understand terms that you are going to find as you go about learning this diet.

- Keto (Keto diet, ketogenic diet): this is a diet that is going to be high in fat, low in carbs, and moderate protein. It is called the keto diet because it forces your body to go into a state of ketosis.
- Paleo diet: this is a diet that is high in protein, low in carbs, and moderate in fats. It is known as the diet of our ancestors and is sometimes described as the diet that you follow where if you cannot gather it or hunt it, you do not eat it.
- Total carbs and net carbs: net carbs are going to be your total carbs without the fiber. When people tell you how to count carbs, you do not ha have to listen to them because there is no wrong way to count carbs. Count them the way that you think is best for you.
- VLCKD (Very low carb ketogenic diet): this diet is obviously going to focus on very low carbs and is going to mean that the user is normally going to take in about fifty grams of carbs a day.
- Zero carb diet: the keto diet is nothing like the zero carb diets that you may have heard of or tried. If you are following a zero carb keto diet you are probably eating about twenty grams of carbs a day. You are most likely also not eating vegetables or eating them in small amounts. People believe that they are going to lose more weight if they follow a zero carb diet, but sadly, there is no proof that this is actually true.

- Nutritional ketosis: nutritional ketosis is going to be when the ketones for the serum are between 0.5 and 3.0 mM. Do not forget that your body reaches ketosis when your body stops forming glucose and is focusing on the utilization of fat that is inside of your system.

- Ketoacidosis: nutritional ketosis is safe for your body, but if you reach ketoacidosis, then you are going to end up having some pretty serious health issues. If you are an alcoholic or have type one or two diabetes then you are more likely to be at risk for ketoacidosis. Your body is going to have about five times more ketones in your body when you are in ketoacidosis. If you have a health issue, you need to talk to your doctor before you try this diet.

- Exogenous ketones: this is the synthetic ketones and the effects that it has on a person's health is still being studied. Normally exogenous ketones enhance the performance of an athlete or may help with some diseases, but you need to be careful with the products you find that have these ketones because they are being marketed incorrectly.

- Keto flu: when you are first getting used to the keto diet, you may experience what is known as the keto flu. You are not actually sick when you are experiencing this, it is just your body getting used to the fact that you are not taking in as many carbohydrates as you were before. You can easily get over these effects by making sure you keep up your electrolytes.

- Electrolytes: the electrolytes are the potassium, sodium, and magnesium levels that are going to be in your system. They are often overlooked when it comes to low carb diets and you need to ensure that you are managing your electrolytes so that you do not have side effects like the keto flu.

- Fat bomb: another hard part of the diet is to manage your fat so that you are eating healthy fats and not the unhealthy kind, especially if you are new to dieting. Fat bombs are going to be things you eat that are high in fat, and low in carbohydrates and protein. These are all snacks that you can enjoy without worrying if you are breaking your diet or not. Benefits of a fat bomb are:
  - Great party snacks
  - Helping manage healthy fats
  - Snacks for before or after you work out
  - If you are trying to fast from fats

- Fat fast: it is going to take up to four weeks for your body to get used to being on a diet. Keep in mind that before your body is used to this diet, your body is going to be used to getting its energy from glucose. Fat fasting is going to be for those who have reached a place in their weight loss where they are no longer losing weight. During this fast you are going to be getting a great majority of calories from the healthy fat that you take in. if you do this, you do not want to do it for more than five days at a time or else you could end up sending your body into starvation and harming yourself.
- Beta-Hydroxybutryate: BHB is a compound that is dissolved by the liver, the first of your ketones are going to be produced by fasting before you start your diet. You can use the blood ketone meter to measure the BHB that is in your system.
- Insulin resistance: IR is a condition in which your cells are not dealing with the insulin in your body like they are supposed to. When someone is IR then they may end up having high blood sugar or high insulin levels in their blood. If this continues to go untreated, someone can end up having type two diabetes or an autoimmune diabetes that is found in adults.
- Metabolic syndrome: when carbs are overcompenstated for you are going to end up with metabolic syndrome which often times leads to hypertension, cardiovascular diseases and many other health issues.
- Medium chain triglycerides: MCT are the saturated fats that our body is going to easily be able to use. They are mostly found in things like coconut oil and are going to be used differently by our body. The MCT is going to go straight to the liver and be converted into energy.
- Saturated fats: SFA is found in things like eggs, red meats, butter and ghee. They last longer on the shelf and are going to have high smoking points. Many of the oils that are used for cooking are going to be SFA. This is also where most of your fat intake should come from.

# Conclusion

Thank you again for downloading this book!

I hope this book was able to help you to find some new recipes for beef that are going to match your ketogenic lifestyle.

The next step is to start trying these recipes! Hopefully you find something new to enjoy and add to your diet that is not going to be unhealthy and is not going to make it to where you are breaking your diet.

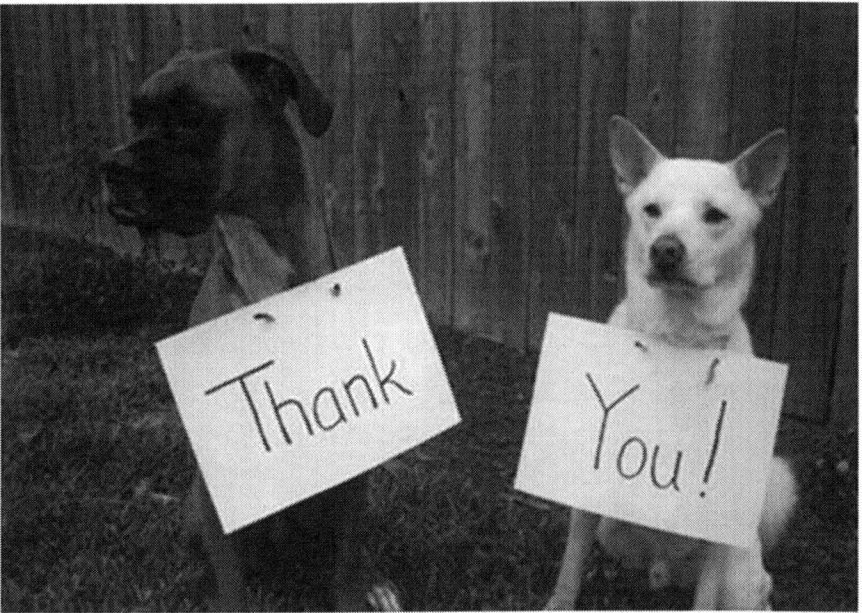

Finally, if you enjoyed this book, then I would like to ask you for a favor, would you be kind enough to leave a review for this book on Amazon? It'd be greatly appreciated!

Click here to leave a review for this book on Amazon!

Thank you and good luck!

# Francesca Bonheur

# *Ketogenic*

# COOKBOOK

RESET YOUR METABOLISM WITH THESE EASY, HEALTHY *and* DELICIOUS KETOGENIC, PALEO *and* PRESSURE COOKER...

VEGAN RECIPES

© Copyright 2017 by Francesca Bonheur - All rights reserved.

The following eBook is reproduced below with the goal of providing information that is as accurate and as reliable as possible. Regardless, purchasing this eBook can be seen as consent to the fact that both the publisher and the author of this book are in no way experts on the topics discussed within, and that any recommendations or suggestions made herein are for entertainment purposes only. Professionals should be consulted as needed before undertaking any of the action endorsed herein.

This declaration is deemed fair and valid by both the American Bar Association and the Committee of Publishers Association and is legally binding throughout the United States.

Furthermore, the transmission, duplication or reproduction of any of the following work, including precise information, will be considered an illegal act, irrespective whether it is done electronically or in print. The legality extends to creating a secondary or tertiary copy of the work or a recorded copy and is only allowed with express written consent of the Publisher. All additional rights are reserved.

The information in the following pages is broadly considered to be a truthful and accurate account of facts, and as such any inattention, use or misuse of the information in question by the reader will render any resulting actions solely under their purview. There are no scenarios in which the publisher or the original author of this work can be in any fashion deemed liable for any hardship or damages that may befall them after undertaking information described herein.

Additionally, the information found on the following pages is intended for informational purposes only and should thus be considered, universal. As befitting its nature, the information presented is without assurance regarding its continued validity or interim quality. Trademarks that mentioned are done without written consent and can in no way be considered an endorsement from the trademark holder.

# Table of Contents

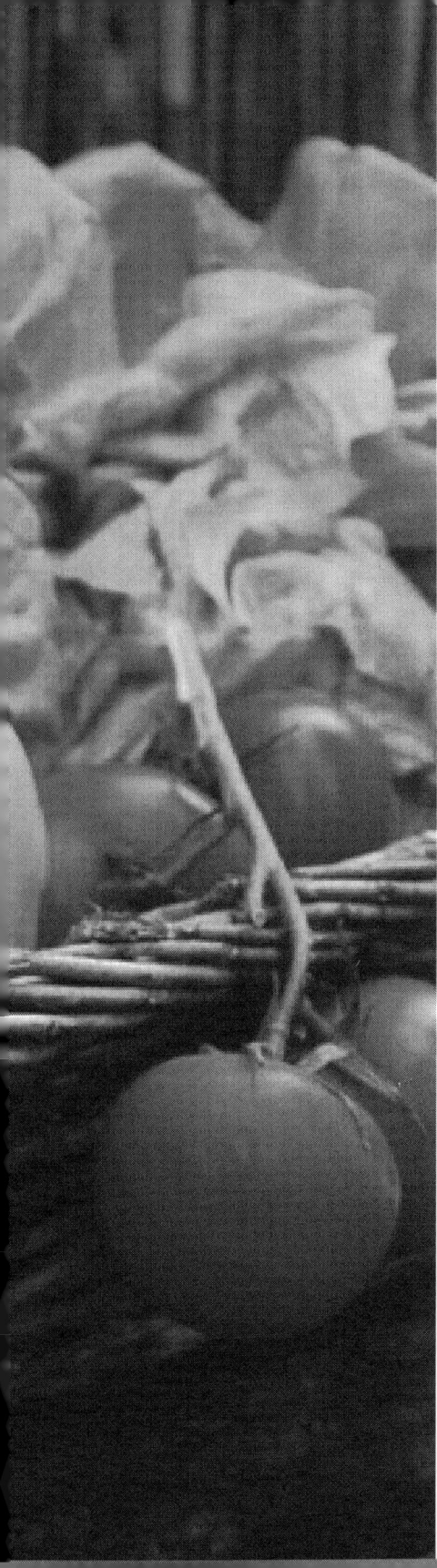

# Introduction

$C$ongratulations on downloading your personal copy of *Ketogenic Cookbook: Reset Your Metabolism with These Easy, Healthy, and Delicious Ketogenic and Pressure Cooker Vegan Recipes*. Thank you for doing so.

The following chapters will discuss some of the many of the benefits of going on the ketogenic diet, such as how it is able to help with many of the health and even neurological disorders that you may be suffering, in addition to helping you to lose that stubborn weight that just won't come off.

You will discover how important it is to work on your health and how the carbs that you are eating now are the downfall to your health. We are going to discuss how the healthy fats that are introduced when eating on the ketogenic diet, and the process of ketosis, will change the way that your body receives its energy and can ensure that you will finally lose some of that weight. Once we understand how great this diet plan can be and all the benefits that come with it, we are going to move on to some great ketogenic and pressure cooker vegan recipes for breakfast lunch, dinner, and snacks. Once we are done, you will be set to get started on the ketogenic diet, even when you are dealing with the vegan lifestyle as well.

There are plenty of books on this subject on the market, thanks again for choosing this one! Every effort was made to ensure it is full of as much useful information as possible. Please enjoy!

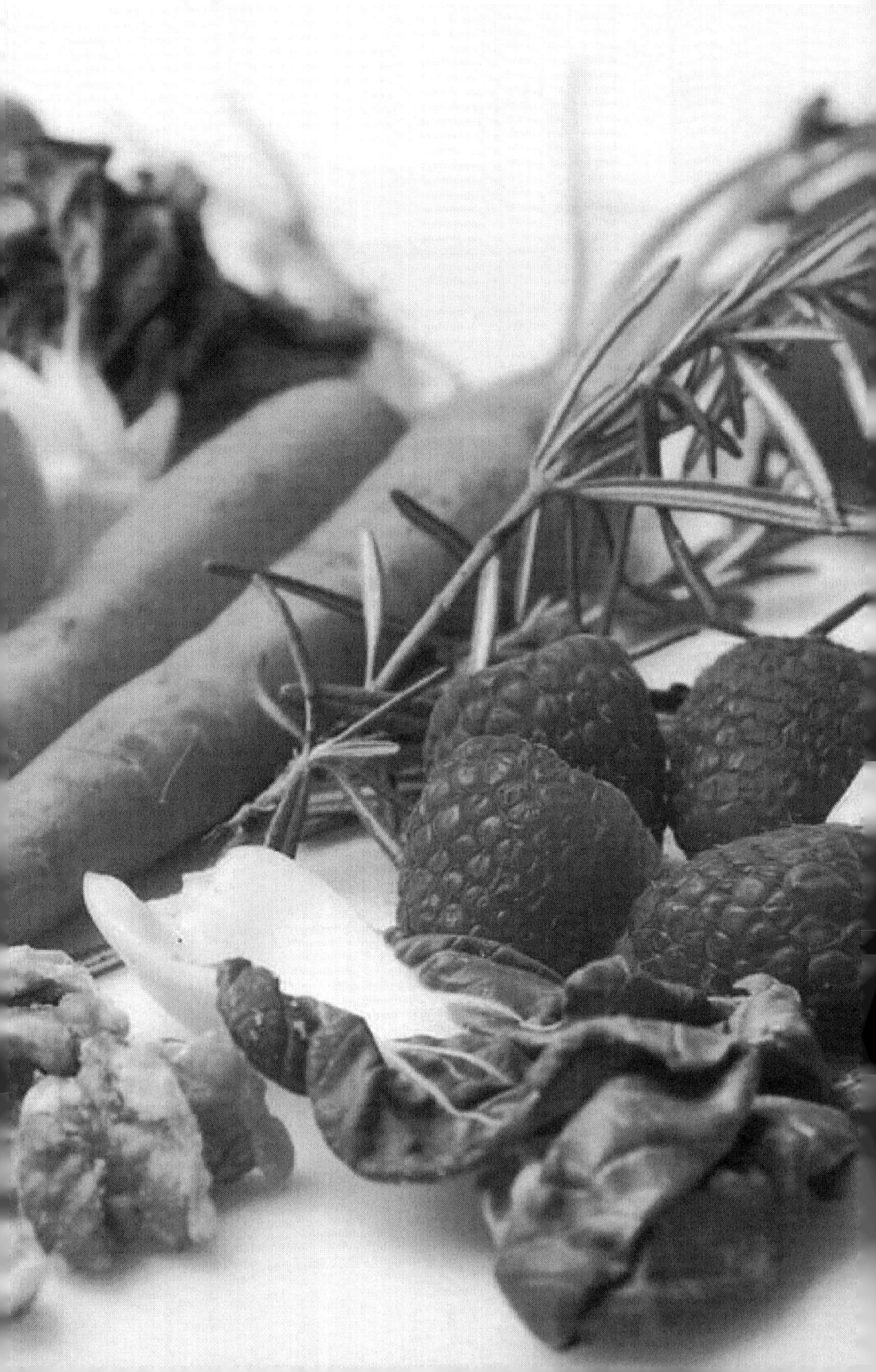

# What is the Ketogenic Diet

The ketogenic diet is unlike the other diet plans that you may try to go on. Most of the traditional diets that Americans choose to go with are full of lots of unhealthy foods that are disguised as healthy foods and can make us sick and keeps the weight stuck on us for the long term. The ketogenic diet will work slightly different, asking you to limit the carbs that you eat, but it is important to remember that not all of the low carb diets that you see are going to be the same as the ketogenic diet. This is because the ketogenic diet has some different rules and while they may seem similar, they are more effective because of some of the changes that come with it for your whole house.

## The basics of ketosis and the ketogenic diet

One of the main components of the ketogenic diet that makes it different than some of the other low carb diets is the process of ketosis. When you are on your typical American diet or one of the other popular diet programs that are out there, you are relying mostly on carbs to provide the body with energy. Whether you eat white and processed carbs or you rely on whole wheat options, carbs are not considered an efficient source of energy.

The body is not going to burn through the carbs as quickly as it should. Often the carbs, unless you are a marathon runner, will go through the digestive system and be converted to sugars inside the body. When combined with other sugars you consume, you could end up with really high blood

3

sugars. This results in a big high for a bit while the body tries to use the energy quickly, but then a big crash is going to follow shortly after.

Once the crash finds you, you will feel hungry and tired and will crave more carbs to keep the body going, even though not all of the carbs from the previous meal have been used up. Throughout the day, you will overeat and never feel full and satisfied and the extra carbs that you are eating (because you will take in more of the carbs and calories than you should) will end up being added fat around the belly.

With the ketogenic diet, you will make some changes to the way that you consume energy for the body. Eating healthy fats is actually the most efficient source of energy. Your body knows how to burn through the fat effectively and you can eat quite a bit of it while still burning through. Many people who eat a ketogenic diet find that they are not only burning through the fat that they eat, but they also burn through a lot of the belly and body fat that has been bothering them for years. You will fell full and satisfied with the foods that are allowed on this diet plan so you won't overeat or feel like you are always hungry, but all that extra energy and the fat burning power is going to make you feel amazing.

Now the process of changing your energy source from carbs over to these healthy fats is known as ketosis. It is going to take a few days for the body to get used to this change and you may feel run down for the first two or three days on the diet. The body is going to search around for the carbs and will be on a low while looking. But it won't take too long before it starts to realize that the carbs are limited and it needs to find an alternate source of energy. With the ketogenic diet, you are limiting the carbs so much that the body is forced to look elsewhere and with all those healthy fats that you will consume, the body will instantly go to these. Once you get past those first few days of low energy, it will all rebound and you will be able to take on any task and enjoy the day more than ever before.

## Why do people choose to go on a ketogenic diet?

With all the different diet plans that are available, you may wonder why so many people would choose an option like the ketogenic diet. What makes this option so much better than all the others. There are many reasons that people would choose this diet type, and weight loss is not the one option. The ketogenic diet was actually introduced as a method for helping cure severe epilepsy in children and then was later adapted to help as a weight loss treatment. Some of the reasons that people are choosing the ketogenic diet rather than another option include:

- Helping to cure severe forms of epilepsy
- Helps with weight reduction in those who are overweight or obese.
- Can help to cure type 2 diabetes by limiting the amounts of sugar in the body.
- Can reduce your risk of heart diseases including helping to change cholesterol levels for the better.
- Helps with other neurological diseases including brain trauma, narcolepsy, Alzheimer's, and Parkinson's.
- Has been shown to help out with those suffering from Polycystic Ovarian Syndrome
- Can help to clear out acne as you get rid of some of the foods that can cause this condition.
- There is emerging evidence that shows how this type of diet is great for dealing with cancer, including brain cancer.
- Some choose to work with this diet plan to help with muscle gain and endurance with weight lifting.

## What would I eat on this diet plan?

So now that we know a bit more about the ketogenic diet and we have some ideas on why it is such a fantastic option to go with, the next question you may have is about eating and the foods allowed on this diet plan. Everyone wants to have an idea of the foods they are allowed to consume and the ones they will need to stick away from in order to see success, to help them determine which diet plan is the best.

Eating on this diet plan is actually quite simple but you do need to be prepared to give up some of the foods that you enjoyed from the past. Some of the rules that come into play when eating on this diet includes the following.

First, we are going to look at the carbs you can consume. The amount of carbs that you consume will determine how quickly, and how long, you will remain in ketosis. Some people are allowed to have more carbs than others, especially those who are intense athletes, while following this plan, but for most individuals, you need to keep your grams of carbs under 60 for the whole day. Those who are trying to deal with their type 2 diabetes or who live a sedentary life may need to go even lower and stick with 30 grams or less. Keep in mind that when you pick out carbs to eat, you should pick options like fruits and vegetables, that have all the nutrition that you need and none of the bad stuff.

Protein is the next nutrient that you should pay attention to. You will not need to eat huge amounts of protein to be on this plan, but you can be a bit higher than the carbs. You will want to aim for between 15 to 20 percent of your calories coming from protein, compared to just 5 percent with the carbs. You should pick out protein sources that are full of the good fats such as ground beef, but having some leaner choices like chicken and fish are great as well on occasion.

The majority of your calories on this plan are going to come from the fat that you eat, somewhere between 75 and 80 percent of them. This does not mean you can go out to your favorite restaurant and eat everything that is deep fried or anything that is in the freezer section of the store. You need to be smart with the fats that you choose and go with options that are healthy, will fill you up, and help you to maintain the energy that you need.

The good news with eating all this fat is that you will gain that extra energy that you need to get through the day and you will actually feel full after a relatively small meal. With your traditional diet, you may eat and eat all day long and still never feel full while gaining weight. But healthy fats are so good for the body and they fill you up, allowing you to not only burn through fat faster in a natural way, but also to reduce the amount of calories that you consume.

## What about being vegan?

The rules that are given above are for those who will follow the traditional form of the ketogenic diet, but what about those who would like to make some modifications to the diet in order to make it vegan? This is something that is allowed as well, you will just need to be a bit careful with your selections.

First we will concentrate on the protein aspect of this. Since most of the traditional forms of protein that people choose would not be allowed on the vegan diet, such as fish, beef, chicken, and eggs, you will not want to consume these. The good news is that protein is a relatively low on the amount of calories that you should consume so you won't have to spend all your time looking for substitutes. You can easily add these in with the help of some of your vegan alternatives to make a tasty meal.

If you are worried about the milk and dairy option, there are plenty of healthy fruits and vegetables that you would be able to consume that contain the same, if not more, of the calcium that you would get from dairy products, so you would simply substitute these out to get the results that you would like.

When it comes to the healthy fats that you will consume on this diet plan, you will easily be able to do this and still remain vegan. Look for healthy oils that are allowed on this diet to cook the food in, go for fruits and vegetables that can add in some of the healthy fats and more. We will provide some great recipes that you can follow in this guidebook while being vegan and on the ketogenic diet so you will find that this is not as impossible as you would think in the beginning.

You may have to make some changes to the diet in order to make it work for being vegan, but it is something that you are able to work with. Just make a few substitutions to the foods that you pick and remember that you need to keep the amounts of macros the right way, and you will be just fine no matter what other dietary needs you have to work with too.

# Ketogenic Vegan Breakfast Meals

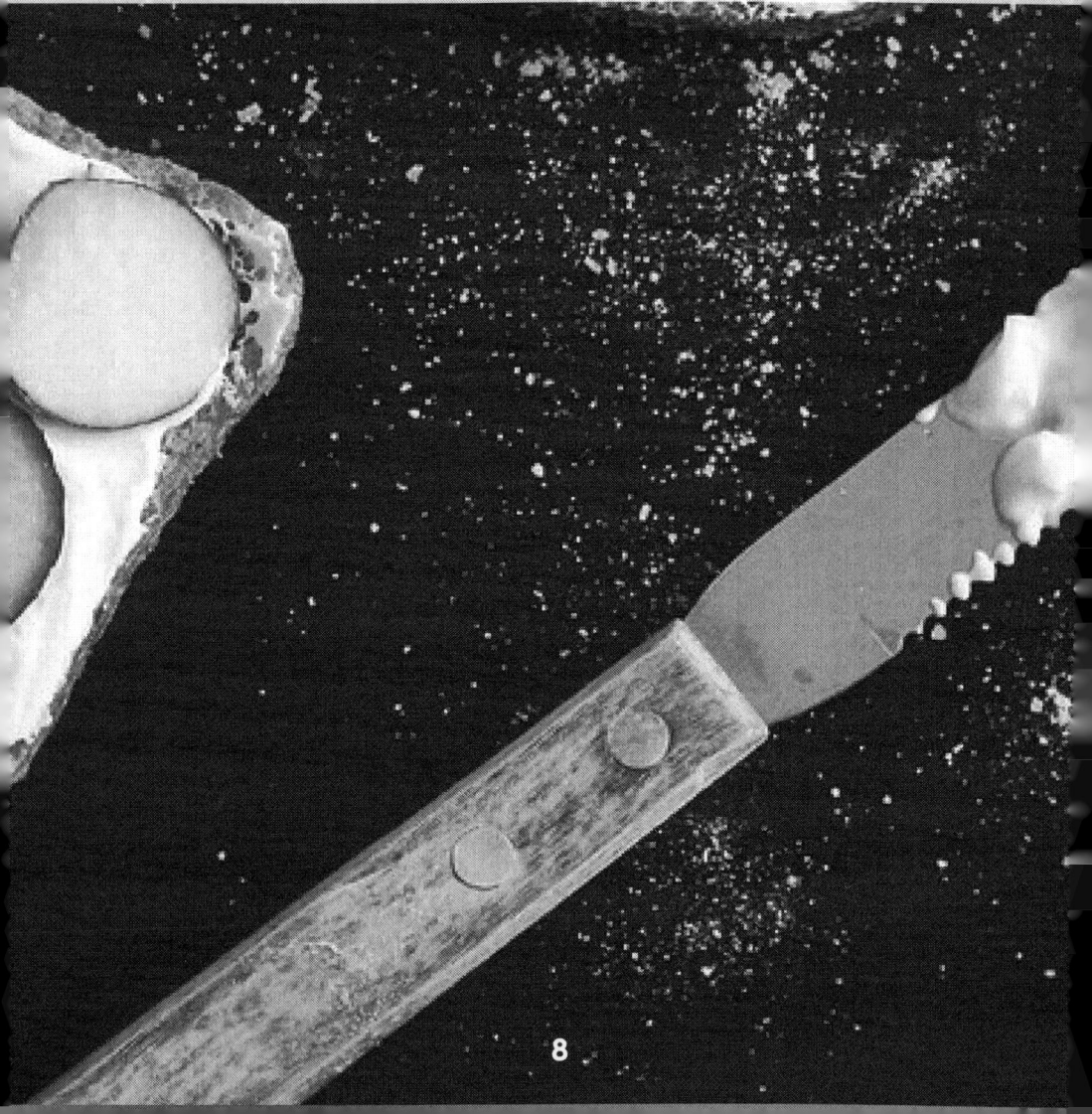

# Breakfast Flatbreads

### Ingredients:

- Water (1/4 c.)
- Baking powder (1/2 tsp.)
- Husk powder (5 Tbsp.)
- Protein powder (1 scoop)
- Cream cheese, non-dairy (6 oz.)
- Blueberries (2 Tbsp.)

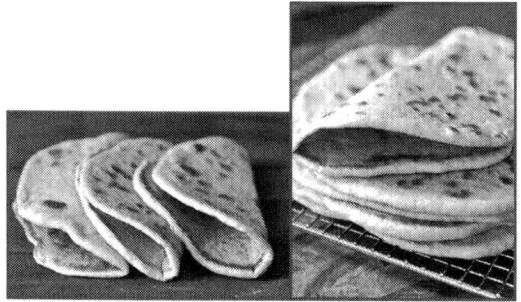

### Directions:

1. Turn on the oven and allow it time to heat until it reaches 350 degrees.

2. Inside a bowl, combine the cheese and an egg replacer together. Place the blueberries into some boiling water to soften a bit.

3. Move the blueberries over and cool down before throwing into the mixture along with the protein powder and husk powder.

4. Allow this to set for a minute to absorb the liquid and mix it well.

5. Take out a baking tray and cover it with the parchment paper. Roll out a bit of this mixture onto the tray and place into the oven. Bake until firm before serving.

# Carrot and Avocado Bowl

## Ingredients:

- Bread
- Cubed tofu (1 c.)
- Tahini (2 Tbsp.)
- Cubed avocado (1)
- Carrots (1/4 c.)
- Dressing
- Lemon juice (1/4 c.)
- Walnuts (2 Tbsp.)
- Salt
- Ginger powder (1 tsp.)
- Olive oil (1/4 c.)
- Poppy seeds (1 Tbsp.)

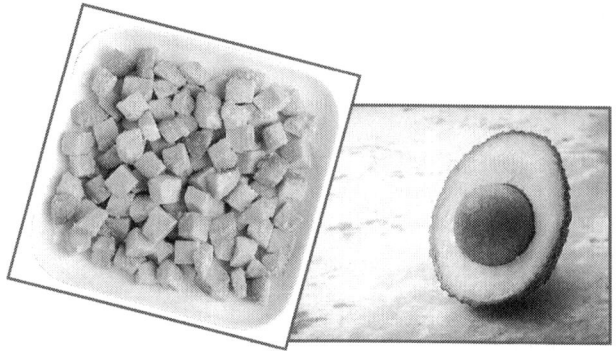

## Directions:

1. Take out a mason jar and pout in the walnuts, salt, lemon juice, olive oil, ginger powder, and poppy seeds. Shake these together well.

2. Inside of a big bowl, place the shredded carrots and cubed avocado. Drizzle the tahini over this before pouring the prepared dressing on top as well.

3. Serve right away.

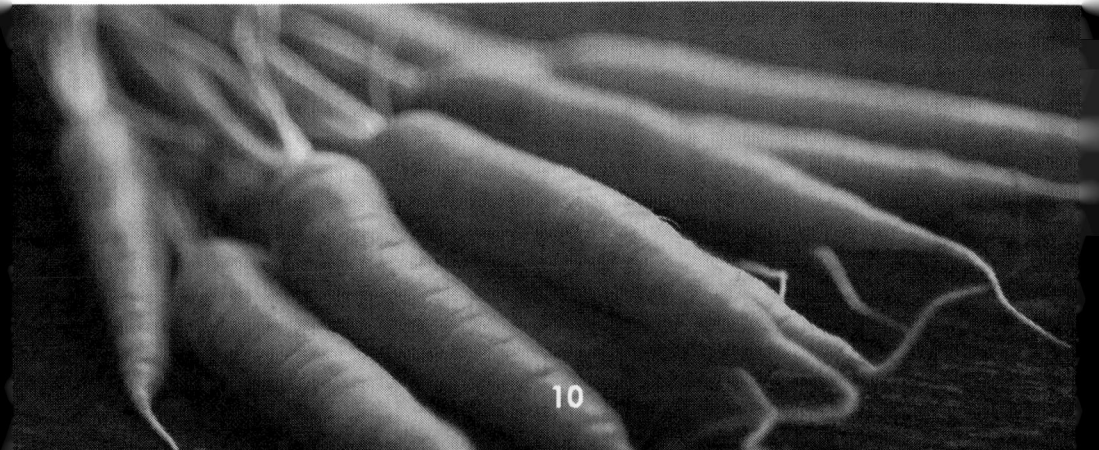

# Healthy Pancakes

### Ingredients:

- Baking powder (1 tsp.)
- Water (1 c.)
- Vanilla (1 tsp.)
- Husk powder (2 Tbsp.)
- Coconut oil (1 Tbsp.)
- Water (1/2 c.)
- Protein powder (2 scoops)
- Almond flour (1/4 c.)

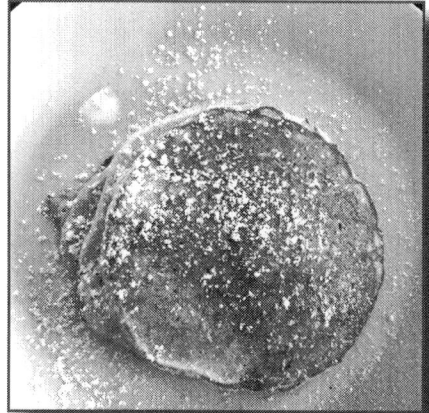

### Directions:

1. Fill up a measuring cup with the ½ cup of water and place the husk powder inside. Let it soak for a bit before removing the water.

2. Add the vanilla as well as the coconut oil.

3. Now combine the dry ingredients together before adding in the rest of the water and mix well.

4. Now slowly add in the protein powder and husk powder in.

5. Heat up a pan. Pour a bit of the batter onto the skillet and let it cook for a bit on one side.

6. When some bubbles start to form on the bottom, flip the pancakes over and then cook a bit longer.

7. Repeat the steps with your remaining batter and then serve.

# Cinnamon Rolls

## Ingredients:

### Filling

➡ Nut butter (1 tsp.)
➡ Cinnamon (2 tsp)
➡ Sweetener, granulated (2 tsp.)
➡ Soy milk (1/4 c.)
➡ Vegan cream cheese (2 Tbsp.)

### Dough

➡ Protein powder (1 ½ scoops)
➡ Baking powder (1 tsp.)
➡ Coconut flour (1/2 c.)
➡ Cinnamon (2 tsp.)
➡ Vegan cream cheese (4 Tbsp.)
➡ Vanilla (1 tsp.)
➡ Water (1/2 c.)
➡ Husk powder (2 Tbsp.)

## Directions:

1. For this recipe, let the oven heat up so that it reaches 350 degrees. Bring out your baking pan and cover with some parchment paper.

2. Place the vanilla and water into a measuring cup and add in the husk powder until it is soft.

3. While that is soaking, take out a bowl and combine the sweetener with the coconut flour, baking powder, and cinnamon.

4. When this is ready, add the husk powder and the cream cheese and then roll the mixture onto the baking pan.

5. Combine your vegan cream cheese, soy milk, sweetener, cinnamon, and nut butter to make the filling and spread this over the dough, leaving a bit of room on the edges.

6. Roll the dough up and place into the fridge to chill a bit.

7. When ready, cut into slices to make the rolls and place onto the baking sheet. You will need to leave these in the oven until the rolls look nice and golden.

# Vegan Keto Porridge

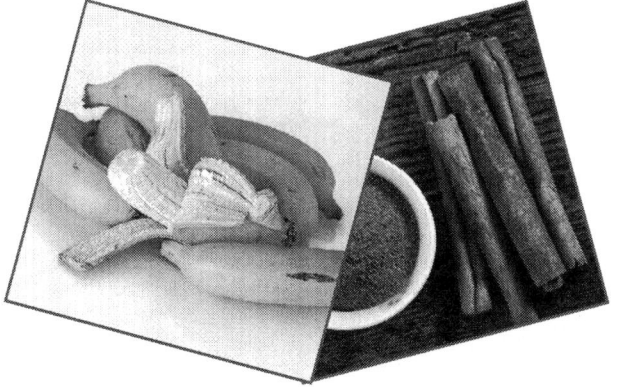

**Ingredients:**

- Cinnamon (dash)
- Bananas (2 sliced)
- Amaranth (1 c.)
- Almond milk (2 ½ c.)

**Directions:**

1. Bring out the pressure cooker and mix together the bananas, amaranth, and milk inside.

2. Place the lid on top to seal and then click on the Manual option. Cook these on the highest pressure for about 3 minutes.

3. When this time is up, press on the cancel button and then allow the pressure to just release all on their own.

4. Serve this with a bit of cinnamon on top and enjoy.

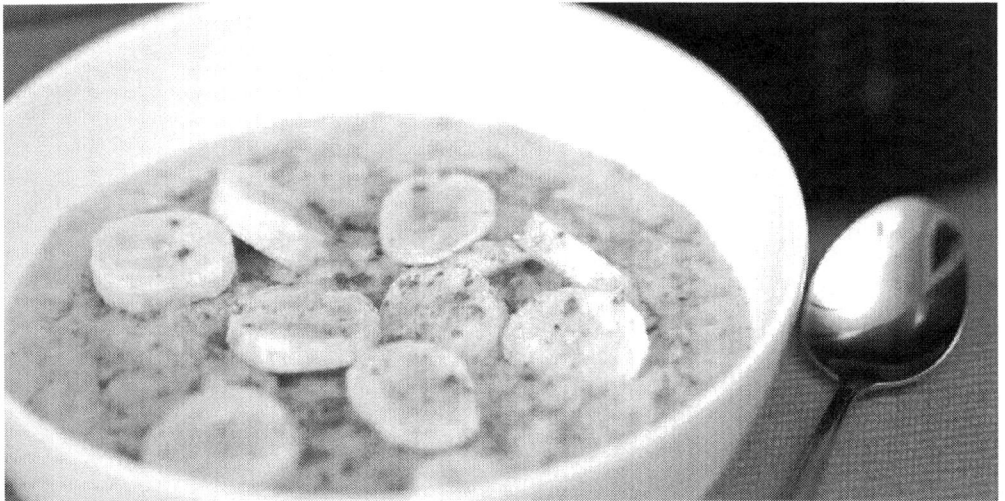

# Sweet Potato Hash

## Ingredients:

→ Hot chili powder (2 tsp.)
→ Chopped sweet potatoes (2 c.)
→ Scallions (1/4 c.)
→ Veggie broth (1/3 c.)
→ Garlic clove (1 minced)
→ Black beans (1 c. cooked)
→ Chopped onion (1 c.)

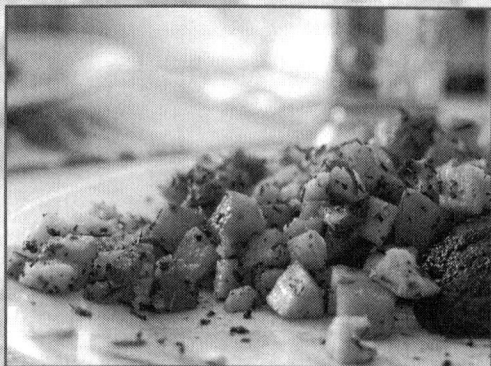

## Directions:

1. Take a bit of time to prep all the vegetables. Turn on your pressure cooker to the saute function and then cook the onion inside for a few minutes, making sure to stir.

2. Now add in the garlic and stir so that these become fragrant together. Throw the chili powder in to coat before adding in the sweet potatoes and the broth.

3. Give these another stir and then lock the lid. Pick the manual pressure and cook this for three minutes to make soft.

4. After these are done cooking, release the pressure a bit and then stir in the scallions and the black beans. Stir to allow everything time to heat up before serving.

# Tofu Scramble

### Ingredients:

- Pepper
- Salt
- Turmeric (1/2 tsp.)
- Dry dill (1 tsp.)
- Diced apple (1)
- Veggie broth (1/4 c.)
- Diced potato (1)
- Garlic cloves (2)
- Onion (1)
- Cherry tomatoes (1 c.)
- Tofu (1 block)

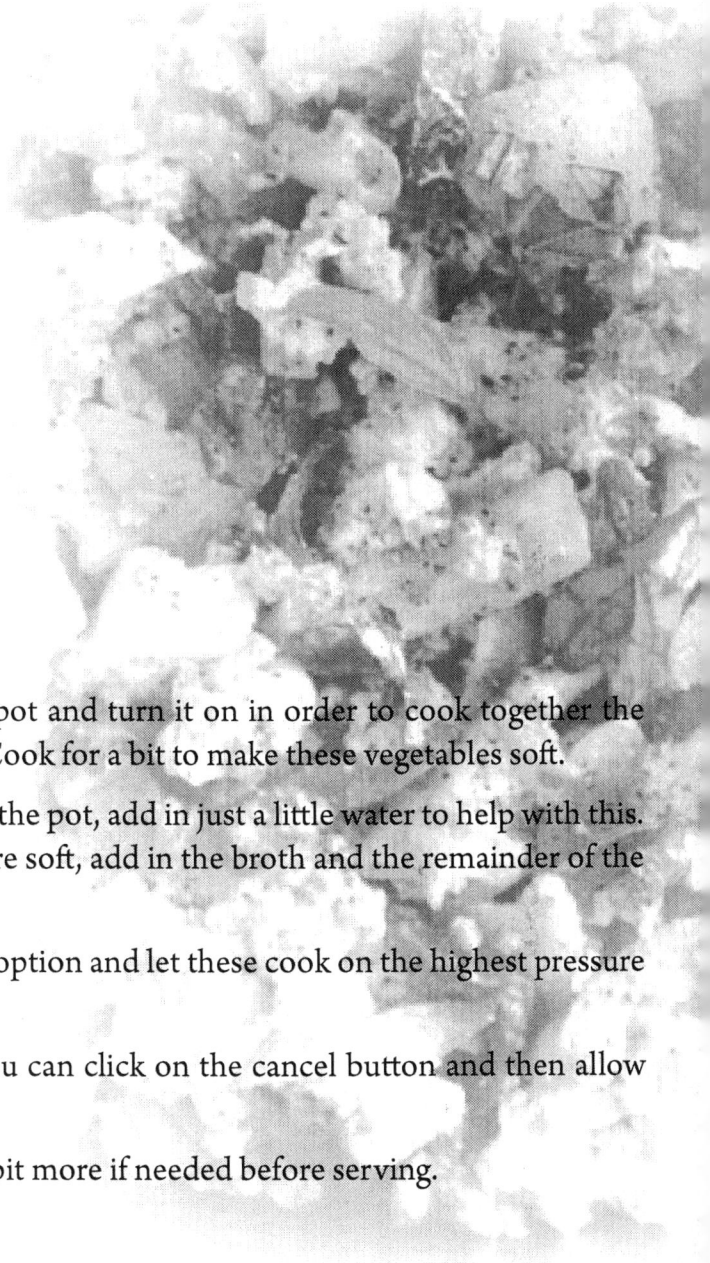

### Directions:

1. Bring out the instant pot and turn it on in order to cook together the onion and the garlic. Cook for a bit to make these vegetables soft.

2. If these are sticking to the pot, add in just a little water to help with this. Once the vegetables are soft, add in the broth and the remainder of the ingredients.

3. Now pick the manual option and let these cook on the highest pressure for 4 to 5 minutes.

4. When this is done, you can click on the cancel button and then allow the pressure out.

5. Stir this and season a bit more if needed before serving.

# Raspberry Swirl

## Ingredients:

### *Swirl*

- Coconut milk (1/4 c.)
- Cream cheese (non-dairy and 1 oz.)

### *Cake*

- Protein powder (1 scoop)
- Vanilla (1 tsp.)
- Baking powder (1 tsp.)
- Egg replacers (4 vegan)
- Cinnamon (1 tsp.)

- Raspberries (1/4 c.)
- Sweetener (2 Tbsp.)
- Non-dairy cream cheese (2 oz.)
- Ground pecans (1 c.)

## Directions:

1. For this recipe, turn the oven so that it reaches 350 degrees.

2. Then find a container and throw in the vegan cream cheese, coconut milk and raspberries into a bowl and set to the side.

3. Inside a blender, add the pecans, egg replacers, vegan cream cheese, sweetener, cinnamon, baking powder, vanilla, and protein powder. Blend these ingredients to make them smooth.

4. Pour the ingredients inside the blender into a prepared cake pan and add in the swirl mixture to the top.

5. This mix needs to end up in your warmed oven and you can allow it to cook until you can insert a fork in the middle and it comes out clean.

6. Take the cake pan out of the oven and give it some time to cool down before you serve.

# Muffin Donuts

## Ingredients:

### Wet ingredients

- Vanilla (1 tsp.)
- Canned coconut milk (1 c.)
- Sweetener (1/4 c.)

### Dry ingredients:

- Salt
- Baking powder (1 tsp.)
- Coconut flour (1/2 c.)
- Nutmeg (1/4 tsp.)
- Protein powder (4 scoops)
- Cinnamon (1 tsp.)

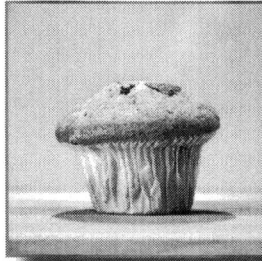

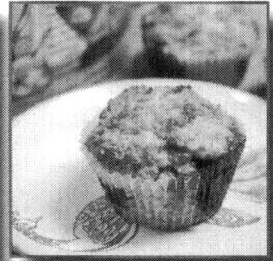

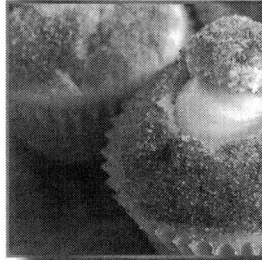

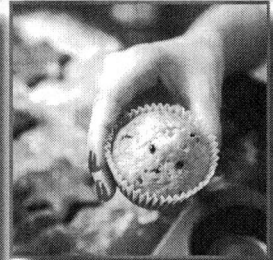

## Directions:

1. With these donuts, turn on your oven so that it can be prepared at 350 degrees. Grease up the muffin tin as well using the cooking spray.

2. Take out a bowl and combine the salt, protein powder, nutmeg, baking powder, coconut flour and cinnamon.

3. Then you will need to bring out a second bowl and place inside the sweetener, vanilla, and the canned coconut milk and mix them well.

4. Take the ingredients that are inside the first bowl and pour them in with the ingredients that are inside the second bowl.

5. Once these are mixed together well without the lumps, pour into the muffin pan, leaving a bit of room on the top.

6. Place into the oven and let them bake for about half an hour before serving.

# Easy Breakfast Bars

## Ingredients:

➡ Protein powder, eggnog flavor (8 scoops)
➡ Sweetener (1/4 c.)
➡ Coffee (1/2 c.)
➡ Soft non-dairy butter (4 Tbsp.)
➡ Vegan cream cheese (5 oz.)

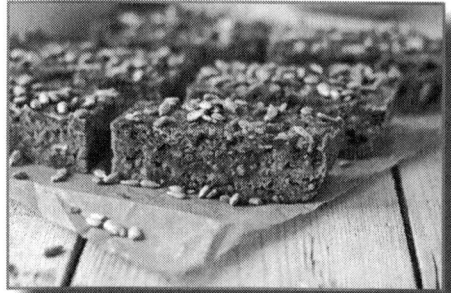

## Directions:

1. To make these breakfast bars, turn on the oven so that it can be prepared at 350 degrees.

2. Inside the first bowl we are going to prepare by creaming the vegan cream cheese, butter, and sugar together.

3. When those have time to be mixed, pour in the coffee and blend some more.

4. Take the 8 scoops of protein powder and add them in as well, stirring in between each of the scoops.

5. Pour this whole thing into your loaf pan before topping with just a dusting of the cinnamon.

6. Place this into the oven and let it go for a bit until they are nice and cooked through before serving.

# Cheesecake Bars

## Ingredients:

- Cinnamon (1 tsp.)
- Coconut flour (2 Tbsp.)
- Protein powder (4 scoops)
- Vanilla protein powder (2 Tbsp.)
- Sweetener (1/4 c.)
- Soft vegan butter (2 Tbsp.)
- Coconut milk (1/2 c.)
- Vegan cream cheese (4 oz.)

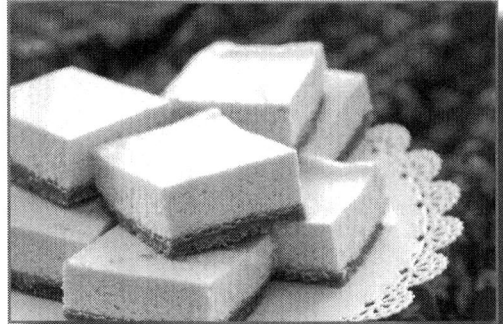

## Directions:

1. To get started with these cheesecake bars, you will need to turn on the oven so that it is ready at 350 degrees.

2. In your first bowl, we are going to get started by blending together the sweetener, butter, and cream cheese.

3. When those have time to mix together, pour in your coconut milk blend a bit more, and then add in the coconut flour and protein powder.

4. When these are blended together well, pour this into a prepared baking pan and sprinkle on a dusting of cinnamon to the top.

5. This dish will need to go inside your hot oven and cook for a bit, usually around 60 minutes. Serve warm.

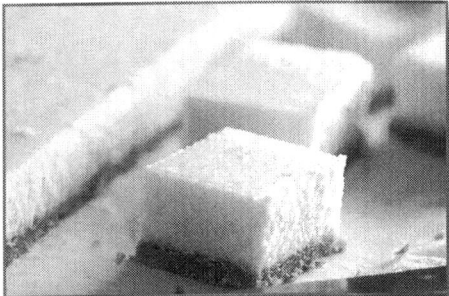

# Berry Bars

## Ingredients:

### Bars

- Sweetener (1/2 c.)
- Chia seeds (2 Tbsp.)
- Vegan milk (3 Tbsp.)
- Salt
- Cinnamon (3/4 tsp.)
- Soft nut butter (1/2 c.)

- Almond flour (2 ¼ c.)
- Vanilla (3/4 tsp.)
- Baking soda (3/4 tsp.)

### Toppings

- Coconut oil (2 Tbsp.)
- Cinnamon (1 tsp.)
- Coconut flakes (1/2 c.)
- Minced pecans (1 c.)
- Strawberry jam (3/4 c.)
- Sweetener (2 Tbsp.)

## Directions:

1. To begin on these berry bars, take out a big bowl and mix up all of your dry ingredients for the bars. You can also turn on the oven and let it heat up to 350 degrees.

2. Now you will need to take some time to add in the wet ingredients well before you throw them in with the dry ingredients.

3. Bring out your big baking pan and cover it all with some parchment paper. Smooth out the bar mixture all over it in an even layer.

4. Top this mixture with the strawberry jam. Now you can work on making the topping. Take out a bowl and throw in all of your ingredients for the topping and drizzle on all over the jam.

5. Place this pan inside of the oven and let it bake for around 20 minutes. Take these bars out of the oven and let them set.

6. Once the bars are at room temperature, place them into the freezer to harden for a few hours before serving.

# Porridge

**Ingredients:**

- Vanilla
- Cinnamon
- Coconut flour (2 Tbsp.)
- Water (1 c.)
- Chia seeds (2 Tbsp.)

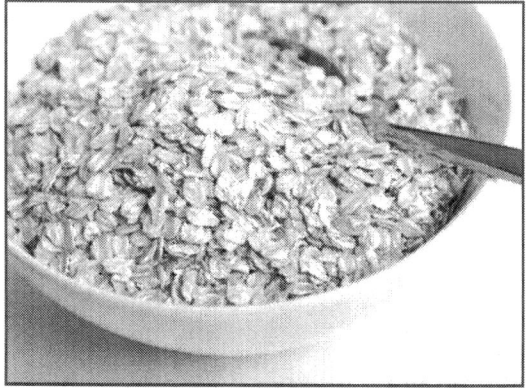

**Directions:**

1. In order to get started with this easy recipe, take out a bowl and just toss all of the ingredients together.

2. After you are done mixing them all together, you can leave them this way for about an hour or eat right away.

3. You can also switch this around for some almond milk instead of water and then add in some more if the consistency is not the right one for you.

# Vanilla Pudding

### Ingredients:

➡ Almonds for topping
➡ Vanilla (1/2 tsp.)
➡ Fruits of your choices for topping
➡ Honey (2 Tbsp.)
➡ Almond milk (2 c.)
➡ Chia seeds (1/2 c.)

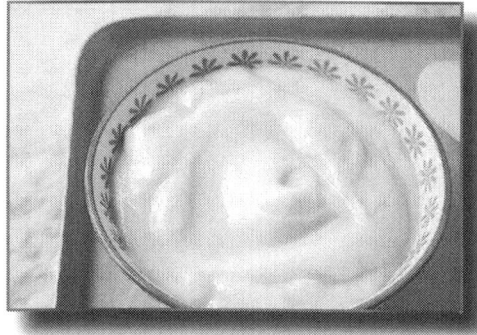

### Directions:

1. To get started on this recipe, you need to find a bit bowl and mix together the vanilla, chia seeds, and the almond milk. You will need to blend the mixture so that it has time to become dense.

2. If you need to, move this over to a bowl that has a lid and then place it into the freezer for a minimum of 1 hour, but preferably for overnight.

3. Before you decide to serve this, make sure to whisk it a bit to make it softer. Pour in some water if it is too dense.

4. When you are ready to serve, place into smaller serving dishes and top with some nuts and fruits of your choices.

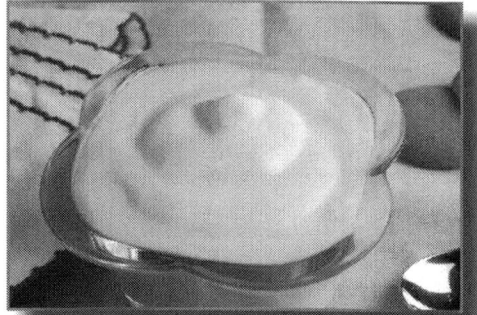

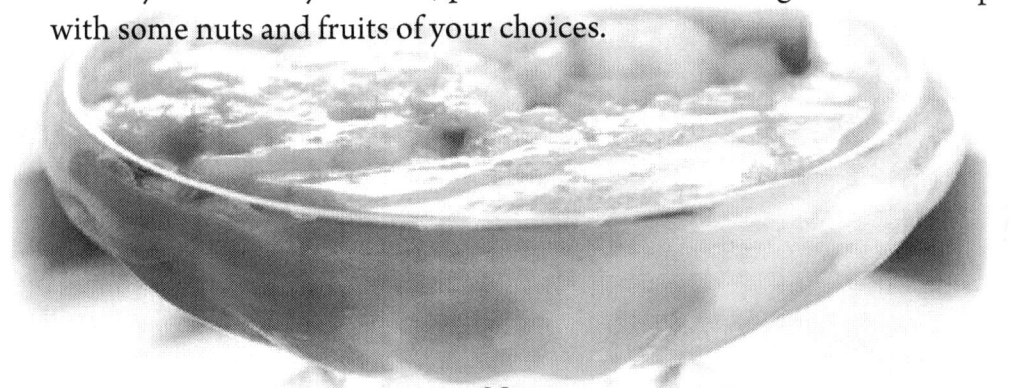

# Vegan Cereal

## Ingredients:

- Cinnamon (1 Tbsp.)
- Maple syrup (1/4 c.)
- Sunflower seeds (1/2 c.)
- Chia seeds (1/4 c.)
- Grated coconut (1 c.)
- Salt
- Soaked chia (1 Tbsp.)

## Directions:

1. To get started for this recipe, take out either a food processor or a blender and jumble together the salt cinnamon, coconut, chia seeds, and sunflower seeds. You will want to blend this until it looks like flour.

2. Place this into a bowl and roll inside the soaked chia and the maple syrup.

3. Delve one scoop of this mixture onto some parchment paper and then top it with another piece.

4. Turn this into a rectangle shape and then discard the upper sheet. When this is ready, slice it into smaller squares, but keep a bit together.

5. Move this piece of paper over to the baking sheet and into your oven, which at this point should be hot at 325 degrees. Bake these until they are a dark brown color. Serve these warm or store them properly.

# Easy Meals to Get Done for Lunch

# Miso Soup

## Ingredients:

- Soy sauce (dash)
- Miso paste (2 Tbsp.)
- Sliced onion (1)
- Chopped carrots (2)
- Silken tofu (1 c.)
- Water (4 c.)

## Directions:

1. For this recipe, bring out the pressure cooker and add in the water, celery, tofu, onion, and carrots inside. Close the lid and get it to seal up well.

2. Push the button for manual and cook this on the highest of the pressures for 6 minutes.

3. Push the button for cancel and then wait a bit so the pressure can get out of the cooker.

4. Open up the lid and then ladle out a bit of the broth. In the both with the broth, add in some miso paste and then whisk to help it dissolve.

5. Pour the miso paste and broth into the pressure cooker and then stir.

6. When it is time to serve, season with just a bit of the soy sauce before serving.

# Winter Vegetable Soup

## Ingredients:

- Chopped celery (1/2 c.)
- Sliced onion (1 c.)
- Parsnip (1 c.)
- Barley (1 c.)
- Vegetable broth (6 c.)
- Carrots (1 ½ c.)
- Winter veggies (2 c.)
- Water (3 c.)
- Pepper
- Salt
- Miso (1 Tbsp. miso with some water)
- Olive oil (1 Tbsp.)
- Tamari (1 Tbsp.)

## Directions:

1. Open up the pressure cooker and push the button to start Sautéing with the oil inside. Add in the onions, carrots, and celery once the oil is warm and brown the vegetables.

2. Now take the broth, barley, tamari, and parsnip inside and then seal up the lid when it is closed.

3. Push on the button to get the manual pressure and then let this cook on a very high pressure for about 8 minutes.

4. Now push on your cancel button and wait a bit so that the pressure can come out of the pot.

5. Dissolve your miso into the water and stir it well into the rest of the dish before serving.

# Root Vegetable Soup

## Ingredients:

- Salt
- Chili powder (1 Tbsp.)
- Vegetable broth (7 c.)
- Garlic powder (2 Tbsp.)
- Coconut oil (1/2 c.)
- Chopped carrots (3 c.)
- Canned tomatoes (1 c.)
- Sweet potatoes (6 c.)

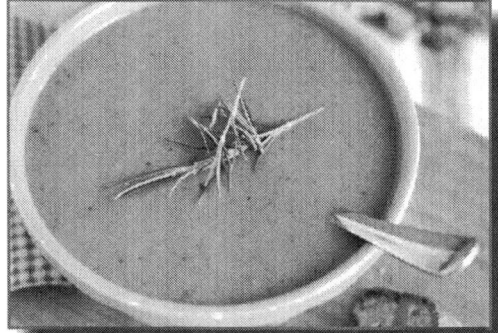

## Directions:

1. Before using the pressure cooker, slice up the potatoes and the carrots and throw them inside. Add in the salt, chili powder, garlic powder, coconut oil, tomatoes, and broth as well.

2. Stir this and put the lid on top to seal. Push the button on the pot for soup and then allow this to cook for half an hour.

3. Now it is time to push the cancel button and then just let the pressure come out for a bit.

4. If you want to make this soup a bit creamier, you can place into the blender so it becomes smooth. Otherwise just serve.

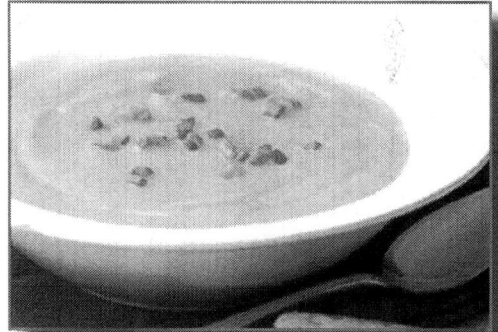

# Guacamole Soup

## Ingredients:

- Small habanero (1/8)
- Oregano (1 tsp.)
- Bay leaf (1)
- Cumin (1 Tbsp.)
- Garlic cloves (3)
- Chopped onion (1)
- Avocados (3 smashed)
- Vegetable stock (4 c.)
- Pepper and salt
- Agave syrup (2 tsp.)

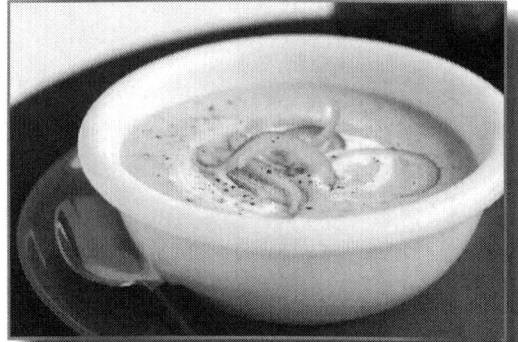

## Directions:

1. Take out the pressure cooker and turn the button on for Sautéing. Now that this pot is warm, place the garlic and onion inside and bake so that they become clear.

2. Now add in the habanero, oregano, bay leaf, cumin, avocados, and vegetable stock and seal the lid on top.

3. Push on the manual button and let this cook on a really high pressure for ten minutes. Then you can press your cancel button and give the pressure time to cool off.

4. Open up the sealed lid and blend the soup in your food processor so it becomes smooth. Add in just a tiny bit of the lime juice and then all the agave syrup before serving.

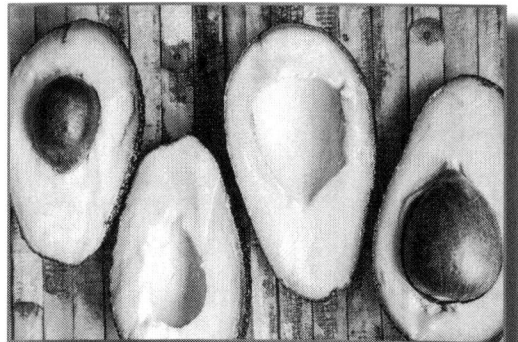

# Spaghetti Squash

### Ingredients:

- Cooked black beans (2 c.)
- Pepper (1/2 tsp.)
- Thyme (1 tsp.)
- Salt
- Rosemary (1 tsp.)
- Parsley (1 tsp.)
- Sage (1/2 tsp.)
- Cooked spaghetti squash (4 c.)
- Olive oil (2 Tbsp.)
- Garlic powder (1 tsp.)

### Directions:

1. To get started with the spaghetti squash, turn on your oven and let it get ready to 350 degrees.

2. Then it is time to prepare the squash. Cut the squash, making sure to take out the seeds, and let it be in half.

3. Place the squash onto a roasting pan, with the slices facing down into the pan, and then let this just sit inside the oven to bake for a bit until soft.

4. After the squash has been in the oven for long enough, it is time to scrape out the flesh.

5. Season this using the spices, herbs, and olive oil that are in the ingredients and mix them together well.

6. Pour this bake into a pan that works well in the oven and put into the oven again for a bit to heat up before serving.

# Cauliflower Nuggets

## Ingredients:

→ Water (1/4 c.)
→ Protein powder (1 scoop)
→ Garbanzo bean flour (1/4 c.)
→ Buffalo wing sauce (2 Tbsp.)
→ Cauliflower florets (2 c.)

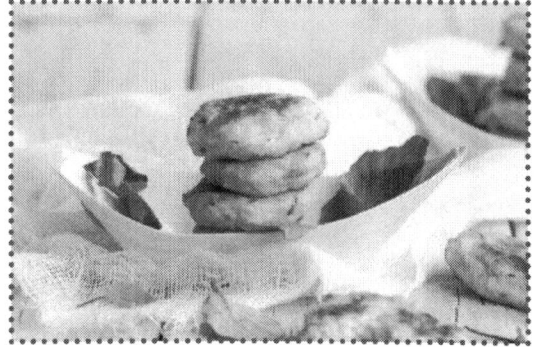

## Directions:

1. To get started with the cauliflower nuggets, you will need to let the oven preheat up to 350 degrees.

2. Cover a baking pan with some cooking spray and then place all of the cauliflower inside. Place into the oven and bake these vegetables for half an hour.

3. While this is cooking, mix together the protein powder, water, chickpea flour, and sauce.

4. When the cauliflower is done, dip each of the pieces into this sauce mixture with your fork before placing all of them back into the baking pan.

5. With the oven still on, put the baking pan back in and allow it to bake for a bit more until nice and ready.

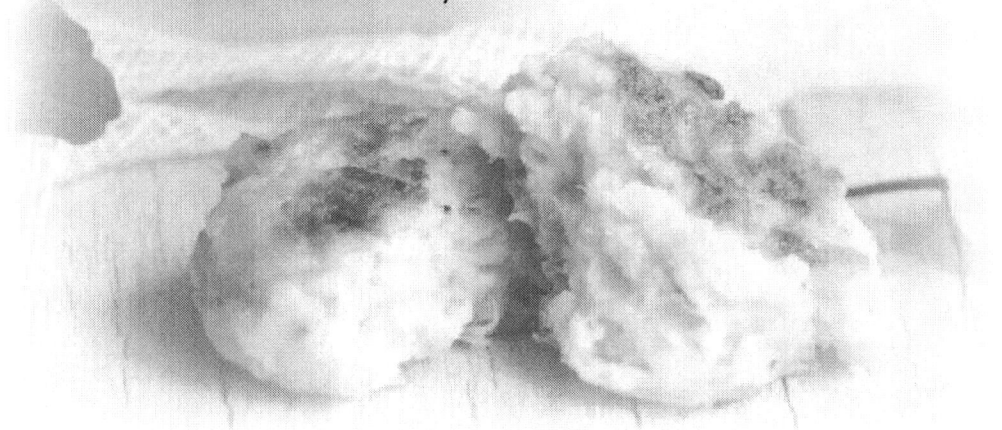

# Lo Mein

## Ingredients:

### Sauce ingredients:

- Chili pepper sauce (1/4 tsp.)
- Tamari (2 Tbsp.)
- Garlic powder (1/2 tsp.)
- Sesame oil (1 Tbsp.)
- Ground ginger (1/2 tsp.)

### Other ingredients:

- Bean sprouts (1/2 c.)
- Shelled edamame (1/2 c.)
- Sliced green beans (1 c.)
- Spinach (1 c.)
- Sliced mushrooms (1/4 c.)
- Julienned carrots (1/4 c.)
- Kelp noodles (1 pack)

## Directions:

1. For this recipe to get started, you will need to take the kelp noodles and let them soak in the water for a while.

2. Then bring out a pan and combine the tamari, garlic powder, ginger, oil, and chili pepper sauce until they are warm.

3. Now you can take the prepared vegetables and throw them in as well, making sure that the bean sprouts go in last of all.

4. Cook these together to make them soft, for around ten minutes, and then add in the kelp noodles that were soaking.

5. Place the lid on top and bring this to a simmer heat for a bit until everything is mixed together well.

# Buffalo Pot Pie

## Ingredients:

### Crust
- Protein powder (2 scoops)
- Vegan egg replacers (2)
- Vegan butter (1/2 c.)
- Coconut flour (3/4 c.)

### Filling
- Vegan shredded cheese (1 c.)
- Buffalo sauce (1/4 c.)
- Chopped cauliflower florets (2 c.)
- Sliced spinach (1/2 c.)

## Directions:

1. In order to begin with this pot pie, you will need to turn on the oven and give it time to reach 350 degrees.

2. Take the cauliflower and lay it out nice and even into your pan then into the oven and let it roast inside for about half an hour.

3. While the cauliflower is being roasted, you can take the vegan butter, coconut flour, egg replacers, and protein powder and combine into a batter.

4. Use your hands to knead this batter. Spread half of it over a baking pie pan of your choice.

5. Then use a container in order t mix the sauce, spinach, and half a cup of cheese together. Put this combination over the pie crust.

6. Take the other half of the dough that you made and place it so that it is on top of the whole dish. Sprinkle on a bit more of the shredded cheese.

7. Now you can place all of the ingredients into the oven and let them bake for half an hour before serving.

# Cheddar Risotto

**Ingredients:**

- Vegan cheese (3 oz.)
- Protein powder (2 scoops)
- Pureed butternut squash (1/2 c.)
- Cauliflower rice (3 c.)
- Diced onion (1 Tbsp.)
- Paprika (2 tsp.)
- Vegan butter (2 Tbsp.)

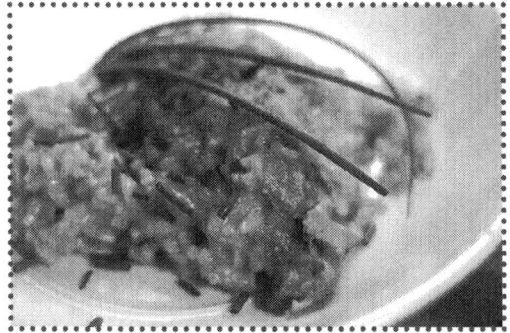

**Directions:**

1. To start the cheddar risotto, take out a pan and melt the butter inside. When the butter starts to get soft, add in the onion and let it cook with the pepper, paprika, and salt.

2. When the onion starts to be kind of see through, add in the protein powder and the prepared butternut squash and mix well before stirring in the cauliflower.

3. Place the lid over this mixture and let it all simmer together, stirring a few times as it goes. You will know that you are done as soon as the cauliflower is looking like rice.

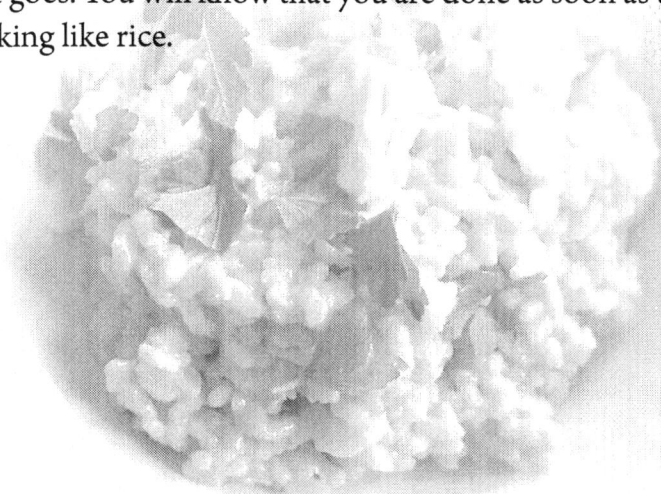

# Cauliflower Garlic Salad

## Ingredients:

- Olive oil (1 Tbsp.)
- Garlic powder (2 tsp.)
- Cauliflower (1)
- Yeast (1 c.)

### Salad

- Spinach (3 handfuls)
- Diced onion (1/2)
- Peeled carrots (3)
- Green peas (1 c.)
- Avocado (1/4)
- Sliced cucumber (1)

## Directions:

1. For this recipe, you will need to take the time to turn the oven up to 375 degrees.

2. When the oven is working on heating up, prepare the vegetables. You can do this by cutting up the cauliflower into florets and grating the carrots.

3. Then take out a bowl and combine the garlic, yeast, and oil. Coat your cauliflower in this mixture before placing into the prepared baking dish.

4. Now throw this into the oven and let the cauliflower go for 60 minutes or until cooked through.

5. When the cauliflower is done, take out a big serving bowl and throw in the carrots, onions, spinach, green peas, avocado and cucumber with the cauliflower and serve.

# Almond Pesto

## Ingredients:

⇒ Walnuts (2 Tbsp.)
⇒ Almonds (2 Tbsp.)
⇒ Spinach (2 c.)
⇒ Arugula leaves (2 c.)
⇒ Garlic clove (1)
⇒ Olive oil (1/2 c.)

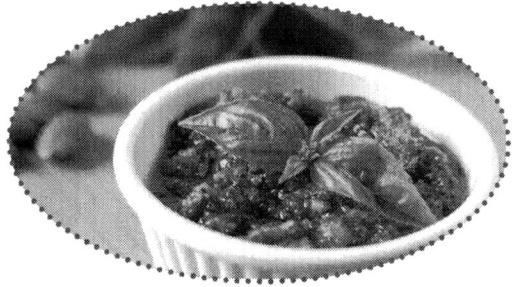

## Directions:

1. When it is time to start the almond pesto, place the garlic, almonds, and walnuts into the food processor and pulverize them.

2. Now add in your spinach, olive oil, and arugula and let this all blend together for a bit longer so that you end up with a nice paste.

3. When this is all done, serve with a bit of spaghetti squash or with some crackers and enjoy.

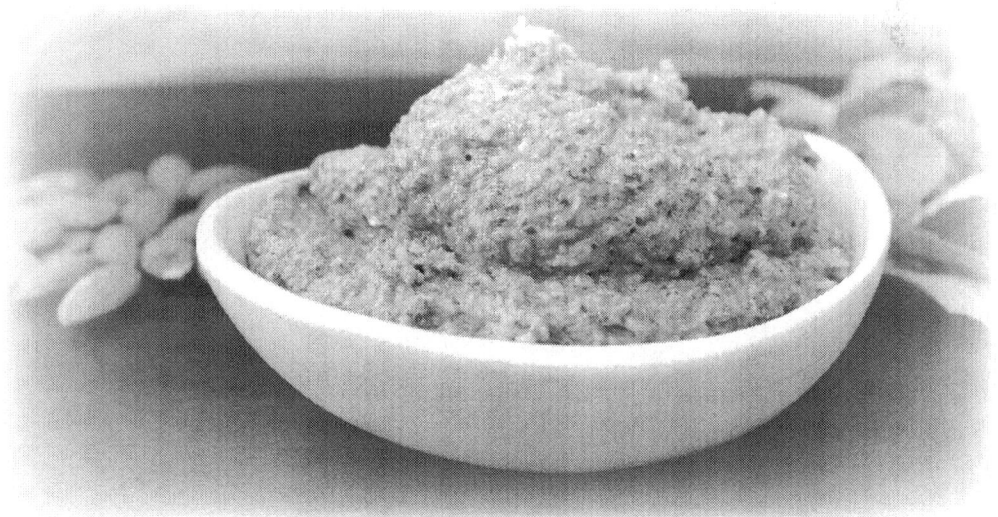

# Cheese and Broccoli Casserole

**Ingredients:**

- Protein powder (3 scoops)
- Vegan egg replacers (8)
- Almond milk (1 c.)
- Vegan cheddar cheese (4 oz.)
- Broccoli (4 c.)

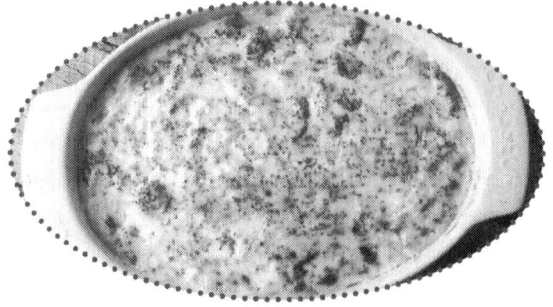

**Directions:**

1. In order to start the cheese and broccoli casserole, you will need to turn on the oven and let it heat up to 350 degrees. Take some parchment paper and use it to line your pie dish.

2. Beat together the eggs and milk until they are smooth before adding in the broccoli and cheese. When this has been seasoned, pour into the prepared pie dish.

3. Sprinkle a bit of cheese over the vegetables and put it into the oven to bake.

4. After half an hour, check the dish and see if it is done before serving.

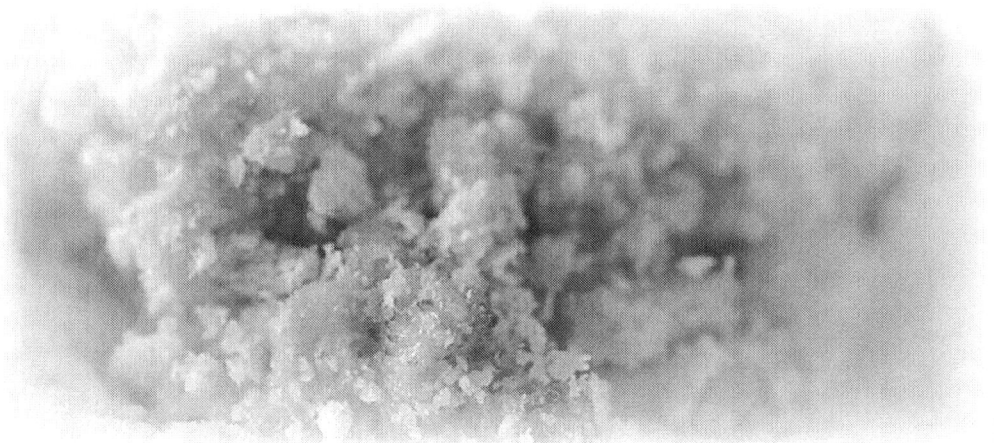

# Dinner Ideas for the Whole Family to be Healthy

# Italian Tofu Scramble

### Ingredients:

- Pepper
- Cumin (1 tsp.)
- Olive oil (1 tsp.)
- Vegetable broth (1/4 c.)
- Italian seasoning (1 Tbsp.)
- Banana pepper rings (2 Tbsp.)
- Diced tomatoes (1 can)
- Firm tofu (1 block)
- Diced carrots (1 c.)
- Sliced onion (1)
- Garlic cloves (3)

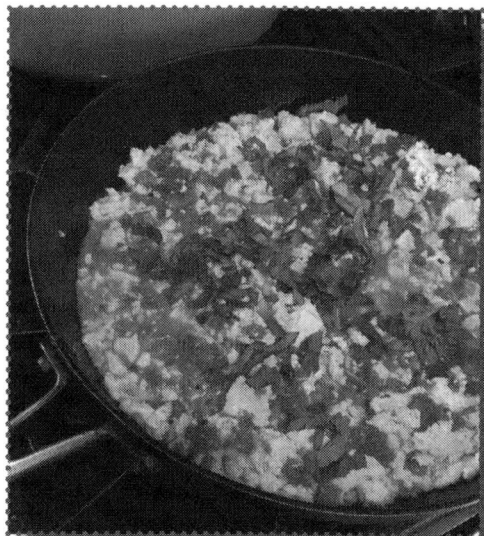

### Directions:

1. Place some of the oil inside your pressure cooker and then press on the button for Sauté.

2. After the oil is able to heat up a bit, add in the carrots, garlic, and onion and let these veggies cook to become soft.

3. Now crumble up the tofu and add it into the pressure cooker with the vegetables. Mix in the seasonings, vegetable broth, tomatoes, and peppers.

4. Seal up the lid of the pressure cooker and then press the button for the manual setting. Cook on a higher pressure for around 4 minutes.

5. Once this time is all done, push on the button for canceling the cooking process and then slowly let the pressure come out before serving.

# Margherita Pizza

## Ingredients:

### Crust
- Protein powder (3 scoops)
- Salt
- Garlic powder (1 tsp.)
- Psyllium powder (2 Tbsp.)
- Baking powder (1 tsp.)
- ground flaxseeds (1/2 c.)
- Vegan cream cheese (1/4 c.)

### Topping
- Vegan cheese (1 c.)
- Chopped basil (1/2 c.)
- Sliced tomato (1)

## Directions:

1. In order to start on the pizza, you will need to turn on the oven and let it heat up to 350 degrees.

2. Take out a pizza pan and line it with some parchment paper.

3. Bring out a bowl and place all of your dry ingredients that are reserved for the crust together before adding the vegan cream cheese.

4. When those are combined a bit, add in the water. Knead this dough a bit before rolling out onto the prepared pizza pan.

5. Place this into the oven and let it cook until the dough is cooked through and brown and then turn it around to bake a bit more on the other side.

6. Top this with the chopped basil and the tomato slices and sprinkle the cheese over it all.

7. Now the pizza will need to go back into the oven for a bit longer until the ingredients are hot and melted and then serve.

# Pad Thai

## Ingredients:

- Walnuts (2 Tbsp.)
- Peanuts (2 Tbsp.)
- Bean sprouts (1 c.)
- Chopped scallion (1 Tbsp.)
- Red pepper flakes (2 tsp.)
- Garlic clove (3)
- Lime juice (1 Tbsp.)
- White onion (1)
- Soy sauce (1/4 c.)
- Peanut butter (1/2 c.)
- Kelp noodles (1 pack)

## Directions:

1. In order to start the pad Thai, bring out a bowl of water and place the kelp noodles inside. Let this soak for a bit.

2. Then you need to take out your food processor and get it all set up, place the garlic, soy sauce, pepper flakes, onion, lime juice, peanuts, peanut butter, and walnuts.

3. Blend these ingredients so that they become nice and smooth and then drain out the noodles.

4. Leave the noodles in a big serving bowl and then pour your sauce so that it is all over it. Add a few scallions on top and then serve!

# Falafel

## Ingredients:

- Salt (1 tsp.)
- Garlic powder (1 tsp.)
- Protein powder (3 scoops)
- All spice (1/4 tsp.)
- Lemon juice (1/4 c.)
- Minced red onion (1/4 c.)
- Parsley (1 tbsp.)
- Cumin (2 tsp.)
- Tahini (1/4 c.)
- Cauliflower rice (1 c.)
- Mixed vegetables (1/3 c.)
- Chickpeas (1 c.)

## Directions:

1. To start off with this recipe, turn on the oven and let it heat up to 350 degrees. Take some parchment paper and line it onto your cookie pan.

2. Now you will need to use your blender and get all of the ingredients inside of it. Allow this to keep on blending until you get a nice paste forming.

3. After this is done, form the paste into some small balls. Place these onto a cookie sheet and into the oven.

4. Bake these for 20 minutes and then serve.

# Mac and Cheese

**Ingredients:**

- Vegan cheese (2 c.)
- Vegan egg replacer (1)
- Protein powder (2 ½ scoops)
- Coconut flour (2 Tbsp.)
- Vegetable broth (1 c.)
- Coconut milk (1 c.
- Cauliflower florets (6 c.)

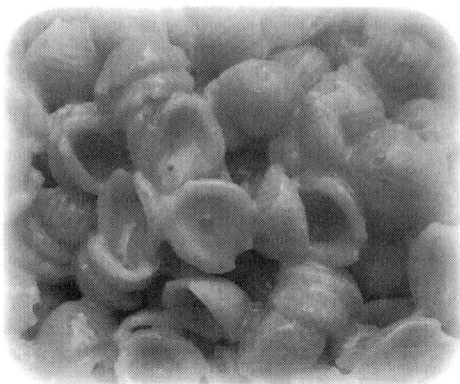

**Directions:**

1. To make the mac and cheese, you will need to turn on the oven and let it get warm to 350 degrees.

2. Now bring out the cauliflower and season it with some salt. Steam this with a double boiler option so that it is cooked through but still a little form.

3. Move these over to your baking pan and set aside. Now you will need to use a pan and warm up the coconut milk before placing the vegetable broth inside.

4. Now you can add in the coconut flour before beating in the vegan egg replacer.

5. After all of this is done, pour the sauce into the baking pan with the cauliflower and then sprinkle your vegan cheese over it all.

6. Place this into the oven and let it cook until everything is bubbly and warm.

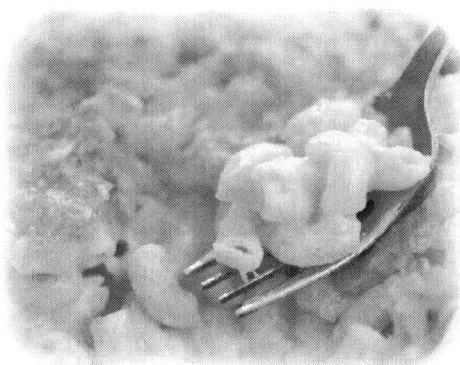

# Potato Soup

**Ingredients:**

- Sliced tofu (1 c.)
- Bay leaf (1)
- Rosemary (1 tsp.)
- Pepper
- Chopped garlic cloves (3)
- Olive oil (1 Tbsp.)
- Coconut milk (1/2 c.)
- Vegetable broth (3 c.)
- Cauliflower rice (3 c.)
- Sliced leek (1)

**Directions:**

1. In order to get started with the potato soup you can bring out your big soup pot and warm up the coconut oil inside.

2. Add the leeks and then let these cook a bit before adding the spices, herbs, garlic, vegetable broth, coconut milk, and cauliflower.

3. Cover the soup pot and let these simmer together until the ingredients are warm and soft.

4. After this time, take the soup from the heat and then blend the mixture inside of a big food processor to make it smooth.

5. Top with the tofu and enjoy.

# Parmesan Eggplant

## Ingredients:

- Olive oil (1/2 c.)
- Protein powder (2 scoops)
- Garlic powder (2 tsp.)
- Almond flour (1 c.)
- Grated vegan cheese (1 c.)
- Salt
- Vegan egg replacer (1)
- Sliced eggplant (1)

## Directions:

1. To start the eggplant meal, we will need to take out a plate and put the eggplant all over it. Season these with some salt and allow them to set for some time.

2. Now you need to take out a small bowl and beat the egg replacer a bit. Then inside another bowl, add in the pepper, cheese, salt, garlic powder, and flour.

3. Take out a big skillet and heat up the oil inside. Dip the prepared slices of eggplant into your vegan egg and then let it get all covered up inside of the flour mixture.

4. Place these covered eggplant slices into the skillet and let them fry until they become browned and crisp.

5. Drain out some of the oil and repeat the process if you still have some of the eggplant left. Serve while these are crispy.

# Mushroom Risotto

## Ingredients:

- Vegan cheese (1/3 c.)
- Vegan butter (4 Tbsp.)
- Chopped chives (3 Tbsp.)
- Vegetable stock (1/4 c.)
- Diced shallots (2)
- Sliced mushrooms (2 lbs.)
- Coconut oil (3 Tbsp.)
- Tofu (3 c.)
- Cauliflower rice (5 c.)

## Directions:

1. In order to start this risotto, you will need to place the tofu and mushrooms onto a skillet and let them cook for a bit to warm up. You can then take them out and place to the side.

2. Now it is time to cook the shallots along with the coconut oil to warm up and then stir in the vegetable broth and cauliflower rice.

3. Keep on simmering this until all of the broth has time to absorb and then take off the stove.

4. Top this skillet mixture with the cheese, tofu, butter, and mushrooms. Season a bit and enjoy.

# Stuffed Eggplant

## Ingredients:

- Cumin (1 tsp.)
- Tomato paste (1 Tbsp.)
- Chopped tomatoes (4)
- Coconut sugar (1 tsp.)
- Chopped parsley (3 Tbsp.)
- Protein powder (2 scoops)
- Chopped green bell pepper (1)
- Chopped onions (2)
- Minced garlic cloves (4)
- Cubed tofu (3 c.)
- Eggplants (6)
- Olive oil (4 Tbsp.)

## Directions:

1. If you would like to get started with the recipe, turn on your oven on so hat it has time to reach 450 degrees. Bring out a baking pan and put a single piece of parchment paper.

2. Slice the eggplant going lengthwise, but don't go all of the way through. Put some salt on the inside and let it set there for a bit.

3. After this time is over, put the eggplant onto your dish and let it go in the oven so everything becomes warm and soft.

4. While your eggplant is cooking, bring out a skillet and warm up the oil with the pepper, onions, and garlic. Let these all cook together until they are soft.

5. Season a bit with the pepper and the salt before adding the tomato, parsley, protein powder, cumin, tomato paste, and sugar.

6. When the eggplants are done cooking, take them out of the oven. Then bring the mixture from the skillet and add it inside the eggplants. Top it all with the tofu cubes.

7. Now take all of the mixture and place it bake into the oven. This is going to need to bake for about 40 minutes and then enjoy.

# Snacks and More for Those Hungry Days

# Mango Chutney

## Ingredients:

- Diced mangos (2)
- Diced apple (1)
- Apple cider vinegar (1 ¼ c.)
- Diced ginger (2 Tbsp.)
- Cinnamon (1/8 tsp.)
- Red pepper flakes (1/2 tsp.)
- Olive oil (1 Tbsp.)
- Cardamom powder (1/4 tsp.)
- Shallot (1)
- Salt (2 tsp.)

## Directions:

1. Take your pressure cooker and turn it on a medium heat to warm up. When it is hot, throw in the shallots as well as the ginger with your oil and cook.

2. Once your shallot becomes soft, add in the cardamom, cinnamon, and chili powder and mix. Throw in everything else at this time.

3. Seal up the lid and click on the manual setting to cook these at a high pressure for seven minutes.

4. Once this is all done, push your cancel button and just let the pressure go out naturally.

5. Push the button for Sauté and leave the lid off. Cook on this setting so the chutney starts to look like jam.

6. Once this dish reaches the texture you would like, ladle this over to glass jars and then close it. Move to the fridge to cool.

# Polenta and Herbs

## Ingredients:

- Rosemary (1 tsp.)
- Minced garlic (2 tsp.)
- Italian parsley (2 Tbsp.)
- Oregano (2 tsp.)
- Basil (3 Tbsp.)
- Bay leaf (1)
- Minced onion (1/2 c.)
- Polenta (1 c.)
- Vegetable broth (4 c.)

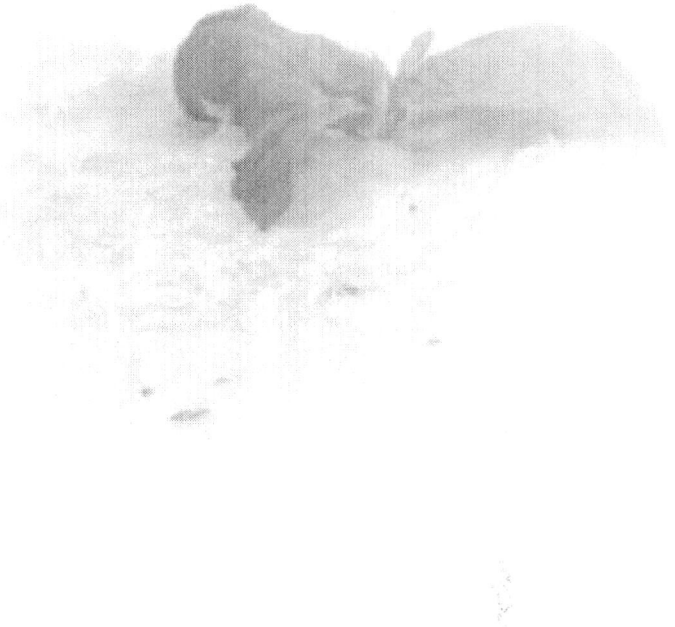

## Directions:

1. Take out the pressure cooker and then dry sauté the onion for a bit. Add in the garlic and cook before adding in the basil, salt, bay leaf, broth, oregano, and rosemary.

2. Stir this around before throwing in the polenta and sealing up the lid.

3. Push on the manual button and then cook this on the highest pressure possible for a bit.

4. When this is all done, push the cancel button and then just let the pressure release as it needs.

5. Use your whisk to stir so that the polenta becomes smooth. If this is too thin for you, simmer a bit longer to make it thicker before serving.

# Porcini Mushroom

### Ingredients:

→ Salt
→ Olive oil (2 Tbsp.)
→ Sliced shallot (1)
→ Dry white wine (1/4 c.)
→ Boiling water (1 c.)
→ Porcini mushrooms (30 g.)
→ Cremini mushrooms (1 lb.)
→ Pepper

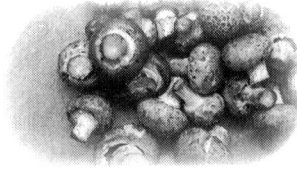

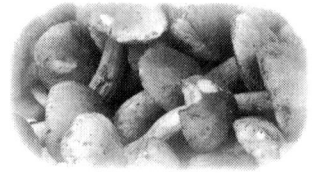

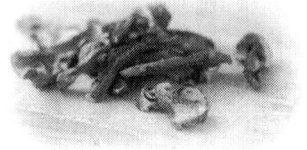

### Directions:

1. Take the porcini mushrooms and place them with the water into a bowl. Cover this whole bowl and then leave it alone for now.

2. Bring out a pressure cooker and heat up some of the oil inside. After this starts to steam, cook the shallot inside.

3. When those are tender, add the cremini mushrooms and allow them to toast. Deglaze this with wine and keep it going until it is all gone.

4. Pour in the water along with the porcini mushrooms and then seal up the lid.

5. Push on the manual button and let this cook on the highest pressure for 10 minutes.

6. Now when that is done, hit the cancel button and let out the pressure quickly. Add in the remainder of the oil and then puree this to make a smooth mixture.

7. Using one of your containers, pour the mixture inside and add on the lid. Leave in the fridge for a bit before you serve.

# Beet Salad and Warm Caper

## Ingredients:

- Pepper
- Chopped parsley (1 Tbsp.)
- Olive oil (1 Tbsp.)
- Salt
- Rice wine vinegar (2 Tbsp.)

- Capers (2 Tbsp.)
- Garlic cloves (1)
- Water (1 c.)
- Beets (4)

## Directions:

1. Bring out the pressure cooker and let it get all set up. Pour in the water and then place in the steamer basket to the pot.

2. Now prepare the beats by cleaning them off and trim them. Set these nicely into the steamer basket and seal up the lid of the pot.

3. Push on the manual button and cook this for a bit, or around 25 minutes.

4. Now when the beat is cooking you will need to work on the dressing. Bring out a Mason jar and place in the capers, salt, oil, pepper, garlic, and parsley and shake well.

5. When the beats are all done, push on the cancel button and then let the pressure out slowly. If the beets are done, you should be able to use a fork to pierce them.

6. Turn on some cold water and then place the beets under while takin the skin off. Slice the beets up and place into a bowl.

7. Top with the jar dressing you just made and then top with the rice wine vinegar before serving.

# Almond cookies

## Ingredients:

- Almond extract (1 tsp.)
- Sunflower oil (2 Tbsp.)
- Almonds (2 c.)
- Water (1 Tbsp.)
- Flax seeds (1/4 c.)
- Vanilla (1 tsp.)
- agave nectar (1/4 c.)
- Baking soda (1/2 tsp.)
- Salt

## Directions:

1. To get started with these cookies, make sure to turn on the oven to 350 degrees. Take some parchment paper and use them to line up two of your cookie sheets.

2. While the oven is getting warm, mix together the flax, salt, almonds, and baking soda inside of your food processor.

3. Keep on mixing this so that this mixture is pretty thick and sticks together once the vanilla and almond extract, agave nectar, and oil are added in. this should start to look like a dough at this time.

4. Roll this dough into balls and then add them to the cookie sheets, making sure to keep them a bit apart. Press them down a little bit.

5. You will need to get these into the oven and let them bake for 10 minutes so the edges look a golden brown, taking the time to rotate around the cookie sheets halfway through the process.

# Almond Brownie Bites

## Ingredients:

- Water (3 Tbsp.)
- Almonds (1 c.)
- Cocoa powder (2 Tbsp.)
- Hemp seeds (1/4 c.)
- Salt
- Olive oil (1 Tbsp.)
- Baking powder (1/2 tsp.)
- Vanilla (2 tsp)
- Baking soda (1/4 tsp.)

## Directions:

1. To start with these brownie bites, turn on the oven and let it heat up to 350 degrees. Use the cocoa to grease up the mini muffin cups that you will use for this.

2. Now take out another bowl and mix the coconut sugar, vanilla, oil, and water and set it to the side.

3. Bring out the food processor and take the baking soda, salt, almonds, baking powder, and hemp seeds inside. Pulse these to make into a smooth powder and then add in your liquid ingredients to make into a dough.

4. Pour this mixture into your prepared muffin cups with the help of a spoon to make them fit well.

5. Get the muffin cups in the oven to bake for a bit. Allow them to just relax and cool down a bit before serving.

# Mustard Green Beans

### Ingredients:

- Raisins (1/4 c.)
- Maple syrup (1 Tbsp.)
- Grainy mustard (1 Tbsp.)
- Olive oil (2 Tbsp.)
- Green beans (1 lb.)
- Balsamic vinegar (1 Tbsp.)
- Chopped pecans (1/4 c.)

### Directions:

1. To start this recipe, bring out a pot and fit it with a steamer basket. Place about an inch of water into the pot before heating this up enough so that it is boiling.

2. Add in the green beans to this mixture and let these cook for 8 minutes so they have time to become tender. When the green beans are nice and soft, place them into a big mixing bowl and set to the side.

3. Now you can bring out another bowl and whisk your olive oil, mustard, agave nectar, and vinegar together.

4. Now take this sauce and place it over the green beans, tossing around to coat well.

5. Throw in the pecans and raisins as well and then serve.

# Energy Muffins

## Ingredients:

- Golden flaxseed meal (2 Tbsp.)
- Almond meal (2 Tbsp.)
- Olive oil (1 tsp.)
- Chica seeds (1 Tbsp.)
- Baking powder (1/2 tsp.)
- Salt

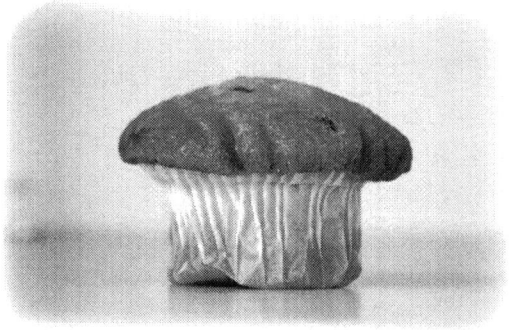

## Directions:

1. In order to get started with this recipe, bring out a mold that will work inside the microwave. Place the flax, almond meal, baking powder, and salt inside.

2. Slowly add in the olive oil (or another type of fat that you would like to use) and mix it well.

3. Place the bowl inside of the microwave and then let these heat up for about a minute before serving.

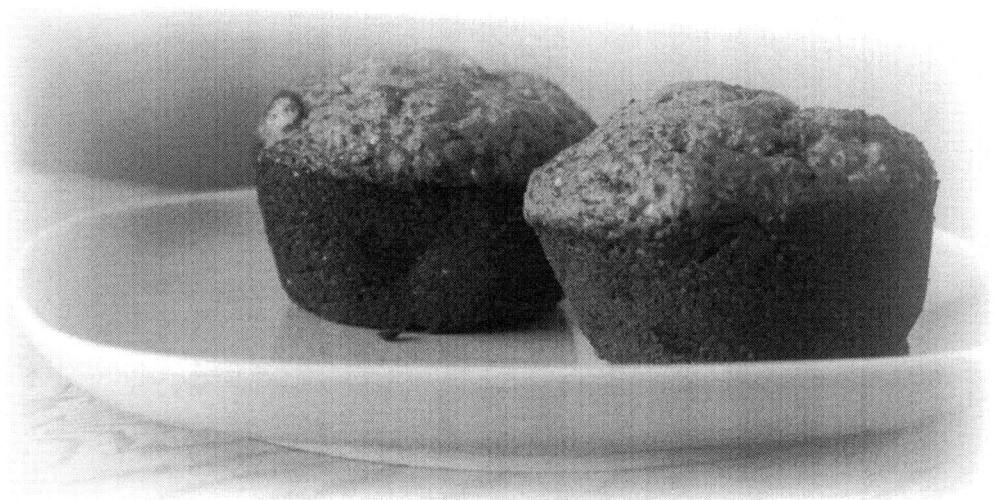

# Japanese Brussel Sprouts

## Ingredients:

- Brussels sprouts (1 lb.)
- Mirin (2 Tbsp.)
- White miso (3 Tbsp.)
- Sesame oil (2 Tbsp.)
- Rice vinegar (1 Tbsp.)
- Ginger syrup (2 Tbsp.)
- Salt

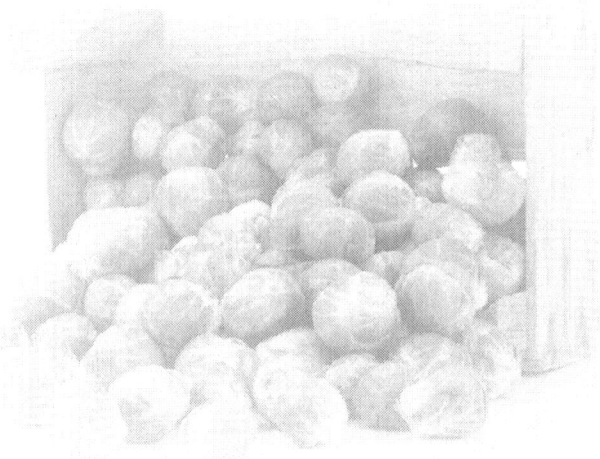

## Directions:

1. For this recipe, turn on the oven and let it get heated up to 400 degrees. Take the time to work on the Brussels sprouts and take all the bad leaves off. Cut your sprouts in half and trim off the stems.

2. Take the sesame oil and spread it out all over a baking sheet that has some parchment paper on it. Sprinkle on the salt and toss around.

3. Lay out the sprouts on the baking pan and place into the oven. You will want to cook these until they become a bright green color.

4. While that sprouts are baking, take out a small bowl and mix the miso, mirin, rice vinegar, and ginger syrup. Take out the sprouts at this time and toss it with the miso glaze.

5. Place this back inside your oven and stir it about three or four times while it is cooking. When these look like they are caramelized and ready to eat, it is time to serve them.

# Pumpkin Muffin

## Ingredients:

- Nutmeg (1/4 tsp.)
- Sweetener (3 Tbsp.)
- Coconut oil (1 Tbsp.)
- Vanilla (1/4 tsp.)
- Apple cider vinegar (1/2 tsp.)
- Cinnamon (1/4 tsp.)
- Baking soda (1/4 tsp.)
- Almond flour (1/4 c.)
- Chia seeds (1 Tbsp.)

## Directions:

1. When you are ready to start this recipe, take out two ramekins and grease them a bit.

2. Then you will need to use a smaller bowl and place all of the ingredients that are dry inside.

3. Then add in all of your other ingredients and take the time to stir them together well.

4. Pour the ingredients all into the ramekins. If you are in a hurry, throw these into the microwave and cook for about 90 seconds. Or if you would like to bake them the longer way in the oven, turn it to warm up to 350 degrees and let these bake 15 minutes.

5. When these are done, take the muffins out of the ramekins and serve them warm.

# Spicy Pasta

## Ingredients:

- Water (1 Tbsp.)
- Minced garlic (1/2 tsp.)
- Ginger (1/2 tsp.)
- Soy sauce (1 ½ tsp.)
- Red pepper flakes (1/8 tsp.)
- Lime juice (1 ½ Tbsp.)
- Sun butter (2 Tbsp.)
- Stevia (5 drops)

*For the noodles*

- Sunflower seeds
- Cucumber (1/2 c.)
- Zucchini (1)
- Carrots (1/4 c.)
- Cilantro (2 Tbsp.)

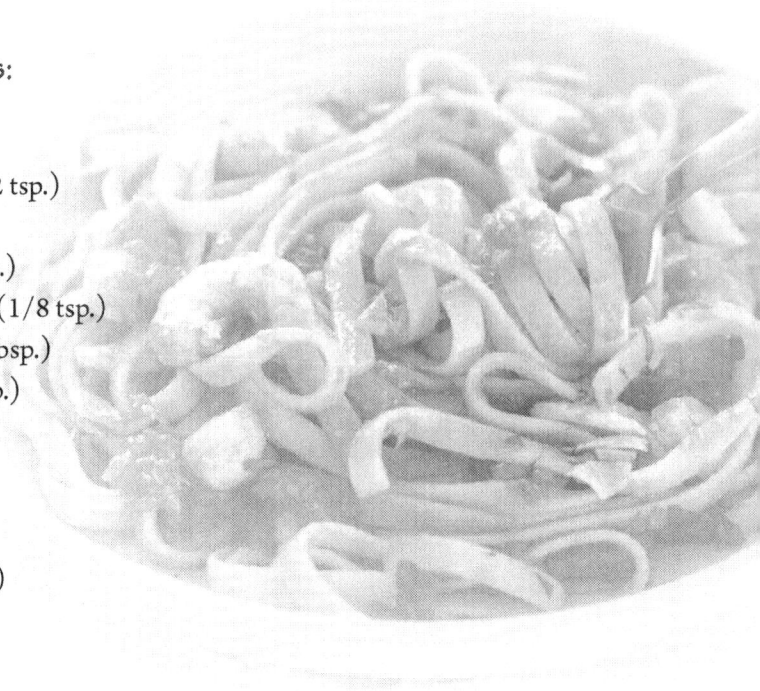

## Directions:

1. For this recipe, you will need to bring out a big blender and place all of your sauce ingredients inside. Combine them until they are done emulsifying.

2. To make the noodles, bring out the spiralizer and prepare the zucchini noodles before sprinkling these with some salt.

3. Place your noodles into a strainer and leave them there for a bit to drain out the water.

4. When you are ready, bring out a big serving bowl and make sure to mix together the sauce and noodles, and the vegetables together. Top with some of the seeds and enjoy.

# Conclusion

Thank for making it through to the end of *Ketogenic Cookbook: Reset Your Metabolism with These Easy, Healthy, and Delicious Ketogenic and Pressure Cooker Vegan Recipes*. Let's hope it was informative and able to provide you with all of the tools you need to achieve your goals of

The next step is to get started on the ketogenic diet. There are many diet plans that you are able to pick from when it comes to working with your health and for those who are on the vegan diet lifestyle, it is even harder to find a diet plan that helps them to be healthy, get the meals done fast, and even helps them to still stick with the vegan lifestyle.

This cookbook is meant to help you to get the results that you would like. We are going to provide you with ketogenic recipes that are all vegan approved to make sticking with both diet plans easier than ever. Add in that many of these recipes can be made using the pressure cooker, a device that can get your meals done in just a few minutes rather than spending hours in the kitchen, and you will find that healthy doesn't mean taking forever.

While this guidebook spends a bit of time talking about the ketogenic diet (and a little bit about how it can be modified for the vegan lifestyle), the main event is all the tasty recipes. We are going to provide you with some great recipes that are easy, healthy, and follow both the ketogenic diet and the vegan diet. From breakfast to lunch to dinner and even snacks, you are going to find the results that you want in no time.

So when you are ready to finally beat through all that bad body fat and the unhealthy life that you are living and you are ready to finally feel healthy and happy, make sure to check out this guidebook and see how easy it can be to stick with your vegan diet while getting all the benefits of the ketogenic diet and creating these meals with the help of the pressure cooker.

Finally, if you found this book useful in any way, a review on Amazon is always appreciated!

# Description

ollowing a healthy diet that is going to make it easier to eat the way that you want while still getting in all of the nutrients that you want. When it comes to working with the ketogenic diet and also staying vegan (while still making sure that the meals are fast and won't take all day) can seem impossible. But this guidebook is going to provide you with all the healthy vegan ketogenic recipes that you need, some of which work with the pressure cooker to get the meal done in just a few minutes, so that you can live the healthy lifestyle that you wish.

Inside this guidebook, you will learn a bit more about the ketogenic diet and how it can work with a vegan lifestyle, along with some of the healthy recipes that you need to make it all work together. Some of the things that you will learn about inside this guidebook include:

- What is the ketogenic diet?
- Easy breakfast meals that are vegan and ketogenic.
- Easy meals to get done for lunch
- Dinner ideas that the whole family will love (and we won't tell them how healthy these diners are)
- And snacks for those days you are really hungry.

Following a vegan ketogenic diet can be a hard thing to do, but with the help of the tips in this guidebook and some of the tasty recipes, and with the help of the pressure cooker, you will be able to make healthy meals that the whole family will love.

43757811R00137

Made in the USA
Middletown, DE
18 May 2017